OXFORD MEDICAL PUBLICATIONS

CLINICAL NEUROSIS

Clinical neurosis

PHILIP SNAITH

Senior Lecturer in Psychiatry
The University of Leeds

OXFORD
OXFORD UNIVERSITY PRESS
NEW YORK   TORONTO
1981

Oxford University Press, Walton Street, Oxford OX2 6DP

OXFORD   LONDON   GLASGOW
NEW YORK   TORONTO   MELBOURNE   WELLINGTON
KUALA LUMPUR   SINGAPORE   JAKARTA   HONG KONG   TOKYO
DELHI   BOMBAY   CALCUTTA   MADRAS   KARACHI
NAIROBI   DAR ES SALAAM   CAPE TOWN

British Library Cataloguing in Publication Data

Snaith, R P
Clinical neurosis.— (Oxford medical publications).
1. Neuroses
I. Title   II. Series
616.8′52   RC 530   80–41212
ISBN 0–19–261251–4

Filmset in Monophoto Times New Roman by
Latimer Trend & Company Ltd Plymouth
Printed in Great Britain by
J. W. Arrowsmith Ltd, Bristol

Contents

Preface

IN 1923 T. A. Ross published *The common neuroses* and this work, with its lucid descriptions of neurotic syndromes, the absence of any of the currently fashionable dogmas, and its broad, humanitarian approach influenced a generation of British psychiatrists. In the United States Laughlin's *The neuroses in clinical practice*, which appeared in 1956, was a larger work than that by Ross. With these exceptions the subject of the neurotic disorders has not achieved the status of the individual textbook and has usually been covered rather summarily in texts of general psychiatry where it is accorded the second-rank status of a shared chapter with disorders of the personality.

With the appearance of Wolpe's *Psychotherapy by reciprocal inhibition* in 1958 there was a surge of interest in the application of the brief psychotherapeutic techniques, known as behaviour therapy, to patients suffering from neurotic disorders. Many teachers and clinicians were doubtful that such an apparently superficial approach could bring about lasting benefit since it was widely believed that the neurotic disorder was the mere external manifestation of a deeper and widespread distortion of the personality and the whole psychic life of the patient. However, accumulating evidence to the contrary is beginning to challenge this prevailing view. Whilst it is accepted that many patients who suffer from neurotic disorders do also have abnormal personality structures this can no longer be held to be invariably the case; in the present book the two concepts of personality disorder and neurotic syndrome have been separated and the latter alone has been fully considered.

At the present time it appears to be worthwhile to assemble the growing number of important reports and studies of neurotic disorders and to attempt a synthesis in a single text. The prime purpose of this text is that of a teaching manual for postgraduate degrees in psychiatry and clinical psychology; however it is recognized that the first and frequently the only clinician to see and treat the neurotic patient is the general practitioner and in many sections of the text the patient's condition has been considered as he first presents in the consulting room of his family doctor.

The book has not attempted to cover such broad themes as the considerations of the basic nature of neurotic disorder or neurosis in relation to the nature of society today. Such themes are essentially speculative areas which still await a consensus on the definition of the concept of neurosis. The topic has therefore been strictly limited to the clinical aspects of neurotic disorder. With the exception of my own area of especial interest in a cognitive-behavioural approach to psychotherapy no attempt has been made to describe other psychotherapeutic techniques for this should only be undertaken by those experienced in them. It was therefore timely that, during the preparation of this book, *An introduction to the psychotherapies* was published, under the editorship of Dr. Sidney Bloch, in which a number of psychotherapeutic techniques were described by acknowledged experts. The student may compensate for the deficiency in the present text by reading Dr. Bloch's book.

The text is divided into chapters which to some extent follow the diagnostic categories of the *International classification of diseases*. However, this is only a device adopted in order to facilitate the assimilation of the material. Neurotic syndromes do not in fact exist in categorical compartments and a greater effort has been expended on the considerations that lead to a formulation of a neurotic disorder than on the narrower diagnostic points by which the particular syndrome shall be recognized. It is hoped that the relatively large list of references appended to each chapter may be of help for those who are planning to undertake research in any particular area. The references which have been asterisked are my own personal choice for seminar reading and other teachers may wish to give priority to the reading list published by the Royal College of Psychiatrists.

Finally I wish to thank Dr. Ian Berg and Dr. Reg Beech who have read sections of the text and offered their own helpful comments. Also I would thank Ray Hanning who, among her other secretarial duties, has undertaken the work of preparation of the manuscript.

Leeds   R. P. Snaith
May 1980

1

Anxiety and the phobic neuroses

PSYCHIATRIC classifications separate anxiety neurosis and phobic neurosis into different categories but this separation is based upon tradition rather than upon clinical realities. Most patients with phobic anxiety, whose anxiety is focussed upon a particular situation, also suffer from some degree of elevation of their general (free-floating) level of anxiety and nearly all patients with generalized anxiety experience an aggravation of their anxiety, often to panic intensity, in some particular situations. Since anxiety neurosis and phobic neurosis do not exist as separate entities they will be considered in the same chapter and the discussion of generalized anxiety will be followed by a more detailed account of phobic anxiety. The consideration of the treatment of all anxiety-based neuroses will be reserved until the end of the chapter.

ANXIETY NEUROSIS

Anxiety is an experience of everyday life which in mild degrees may be serviceable to the individual but in more severe degrees is destructive. It is both a spur to action and a hindrance to effective performance; it is willingly sought by those who engage in dangerous sport and by those who watch them for the vicarious thrill; the neurotic patient will attempt to avoid anxiety at the cost of severe handicap of his life style. Lewis (1970), in his consideration of the ambiguous word, anxiety, listed among the technical and clinical applications of the word:

    1. An emotional state with the subjectively experienced quality of fear;

    2. An unpleasant emotion which may be accompanied by a feeling of impending death;

    3. Anxiety is directed to the future, implicit in the feeling that there is a threat of some kind;

    4. There may be no recognizable threat or one which, by

reasonable standards, is out of proportion to the emotion it seemingly provokes;

5. There may be subjective bodily discomfort and manifest bodily disturbance.

Many profound works have considered the nature of normal anxiety but in this present chapter the topic will be circumscribed to morbid, or clinical, anxiety. The work *Clinical anxiety* (Lader and Marks, 1971) covers the subject in its wider aspect.

Anxiety must be considered under the two concepts of trait anxiety and state anxiety. The former refers to an enduring aspect of the personality structure and the latter to a temporal disorder. There is an increasing tendency to use the term anxiety state rather than the term anxiety neurosis. This arises from the attempt to avoid the ambiguities of the 9th Revision of the *International classification of diseases* where there is no separate category in the section on 'personality disorder' for the individual with severe trait anxiety and where the term 'anxiety neurosis', as defined in the Glossary (1978) may serve for both trait and state:

> Anxiety neurosis. Includes various combinations of physical and mental manifestations of anxiety not attributed to real danger and occurring either in attacks or as a persisting state. The anxiety is usually diffuse and may extend to panic. Other neurotic features, such as obsessional or hysterical symptoms, may be present but do not dominate the clinical picture.

However, with the introduction of more effective treatment, it is necessary to distinguish trait anxiety from state anxiety, whilst recognizing that they often occur together, for the management of the two forms will be different.

Trait anxiety may be partly genetically determined and partly the outcome of early experience of the individual. The evidence for the genetic basis has been reviewed by Young, Fenton, and Lader (1971) who, in their own study, confirmed the presence of this factor. State anxiety may result from stress or conflict which may be acute or prolonged, or it may arise in the absence of any sufficient stress to account for it; in the latter case its basis is usually that of an endogenous affective disorder. State anxiety may also result from certain physiological and pathological processes such as premenstrual tension, disease of the limbic structures of the brain, thyrotoxicosis, or tumours of the adrenal gland leading to an overproduction of adrenaline. It may result from the ingestion of large amounts of caffeine from excessive tea or coffee drinking, or other drugs such as amphetamine.

Anxiety may be experienced entirely as psychic discomfort characterized by the symptoms of apprehension, diffuse fear, and, in its most severe degree, panic. However it may be partly somatized and somatic symptoms may dominate the picture; among the wide variety of somatic symptoms are muscular pains, tension headache, tremor, palpitations, diarrhoea, sweating, respiratory distress, feelings of dizziness, swaying, and 'walking on cotton wool'. In mild degree anxiety may be no more than a slight awareness of discomfort but the most severe degree was graphically described in the seventeenth century by Robert Burton in *The anatomy of melancholy*:

> Many men are so amazed and astonished with fear that they know not where they are, what they say, what they do, and that which is worst, it tortures them many days before with continual affrights and suspicion. It hinders most honourable attempts, and makes their hearts ache, sad and heavy. They that live in fear are never free, resolute, secure or merry but in continual pain; that, as Vives truly said, no greater misery, no rack, no torture like unto it.

Some of the variety of combinations of trait and state anxiety will now be clarified by means of brief clinical examples.

Trait anxiety. John was 16 when he was referred to an adolescent unit on account of headaches, insomnia, and a marked reluctance to engage in any type of social activity. Throughout his life he had been a tense, retiring child, nervous of the possibility of any type of injury, and he had played with few other children. His mother was an unhappy person who had consumed large amounts of sedative drugs for many years. John's birth had been premature and he was raised in an atmosphere of parental solicitude, being kept at home for every trivial ill and injury.

State anxiety on the basis of trait anxiety. At the age of 25 Jane became generally anxious following a minor traffic accident during which there had been no physical injury to herself or others. Four months after the accident she was still awaking from anxiety dreams, and during the day she experienced a pervasive foreboding of disaster, had difficulty in concentrating and was losing weight. She was an efficient secretary but was making an increasing number of mistakes and her boss advised her to see a doctor. She was at a loss to account for feeling so anxious after such slight trauma.

A careful history was supplemented by an account from her parents who recalled that Jane had been tense and fearful as a child but had always admired courage; a picture of Grace Darling hung on her nursery wall. She set herself the task of overcoming her timidity by joining groups of adventurous youngsters and by the age of 10 she had largely succeeded in the task of masking her trait anxiety with a facade of boldness. The recent accident had wounded her in her Achilles heel.

State anxiety resembling trait anxiety. Jack was 30 when his general practitioner considered he was requesting too many sedative and analgesic drugs for insomnia and vague bodily aches and pains. He arranged to see him at a long interview. Jack accepted that he 'was some sort of a nervous case' and described periodic anxiety attacks and a constant difficulty in relaxing; he admitted that he was irritable and that his wife had threatened to leave on account of this. When asked about the onset of these symptoms he replied that he had always had them. He agreed to his mother being interviewed.

His mother stated that Jack had been 'a perfectly normal, lively youngster and as fearless as the rest of his playmates' but when he was eight years old his father left the home and they subsequently divorced. Jack had admired his father and was perplexed about the desertion. He lost his appetite and although he improved he never seemed to regain his carefree spirit. Difficult home circumstances had perpetuated the anxiety. Although the anxiety was longstanding it was nevertheless a chronic state anxiety, having a definite onset in time.

State anxiety (endogenous). Joan was 38 years old when she first began to feel uneasy in crowds; she also began to sleep badly and suffered an oppressive sense of constriction in her chest. She felt tense and had difficulty in relaxing. About three weeks after the onset of these symptoms she had a panic attack in a supermarket and from that time her activities were progressively restricted by anxiety; she did not like to walk more than a few yards from her home and the anticipation of further panic made it impossible for her to travel by bus or enter large shops. All her early symptoms worsened.

Joan was unable to account for the onset of her anxiety and could only recall that an aunt had died some weeks before but the death had been expected and she was not severely upset on receipt of the news. Careful enquiry from Joan and her husband did not reveal any precipitant or stress adequate to account for such severe and persisting anxiety. Her mental and physical health had always been good although she recalled that, as a child, she sometimes felt faint during the school morning assembly. Her personality structure was not abnormal by reason of any undue degree of an adverse trait but she considered that she was rather more punctilious and houseproud than most women she knew. At the age of 50 her father had been treated with ECT for a depressive illness.

The above examples illustrate some of the ways in which anxiety may present in clinical practice but there are an infinite number of variations. Most simple anxiety neuroses can be understood in terms of external stress acting upon a susceptible personality but many of the more severe states are in fact a form of affective disorder for which this simple model does not provide an adequate explanation. Most writers on the subject have tended to assume that anxiety neurosis is a homogeneous entity rather than a spectrum of disorders; as a result there have been unfortunate attempts to force all anxiety neuroses, Procrustean fashion, into some single theoretical explanation. Kraüpl Taylor (1966) is among those who have recognized the fallacy of such attempts and has pointed out that if anxiety-dominated neuroses develop in the absence of any recognizable psychogenic trauma, traumatization is then assumed to have occurred so long ago that it has become 'unconscious': 'The pursuit of presumed traumatic experiences is forced further and further back to the earliest days of the individual's postnatal existence until the decision can no longer be avoided whether to admit a hereditary determination of psychogenic reactivity, or to postulate that the event of being born was the first pathogenic experience.'

Anxiety, depression, and affective disorder

The nosological status of anxiety neurosis has always been insecure and, as with the distinction between neurotic and psychotic depressive states which is considered in the next chapter, psychiatrists are divided into two broad and conflicting camps; the separatists hold the view that anxiety and depressive disorders are basically separate conditions but the opposing group, the dimensionalists, consider that there is no absolute separation but rather a continuum of mood disturbance from anxiety, through 'anxiety-depression' in equal proportions to depression. This latter view has been supported by Mapother (1926) and by Lewis (1966) who wrote that affective disorders could be divided into three broad groups, each with a major and a minor variant: agitated depression and anxiety state; retarded depression and mild, neurasthenic depression; mania and hypomania. Garmany (1956) is usually quoted as representing the separatist view but nevertheless he pointed out that: 'Most acute anxiety states referred urgently to hospital turn out to be suffering from depression.'

The feasibility of a true distinction between anxiety states and depressive illness will be considered in three broad areas: clinical features during the key illness; outcome studies; treatment studies.

Clinical features

In 1972 Roth and his colleagues in Newcastle upon Tyne published a series of four studies upholding the view that there is a true distinction between anxiety states and depressive disorder. In the first two of these papers (Roth *et al.*, 1972; Gurney *et al.*, 1972) they examined a number of items drawn from the early life, personality, and clinical features of two groups of patients, one group diagnosed as suffering from anxiety state and the other from depressive illness. These patients were all in-patients and so, especially in the case of the anxiety group, may not have been truly representative of the category as a whole. The conclusion was drawn from the data that there is a true distinction to be found between the two disorders but the certainty of this conclusion is reduced by the possibility, recognized by the authors, that observer bias may have affected the recording of the data; this methodological fault will be more fully expanded in Chapter 2.

Scales completed by the patient, although subject to their own source of error, will be free from influence by the theoretical views of the research psychiatrist and it may be expected that investigations based upon this technique would confirm or reject the conclusions of other types of enquiry. One such investigation was carried out by Prusoff and Klerman (1974) on a large number of female out-patients diagnosed as suffering either from anxiety neurosis or from neurotic depression; they used a rather large 58-item self-report questionnaire, the Symptom Check List, which divided up into five main areas of symptomatology: somatic symptoms, obsessions, interpersonal relationships, anxiety, and depression. Apart from the somatic scale they found that the depressed patients recorded themselves as being more severely disturbed on all the scales including the anxiety scale and they found an unsatisfactory degree of separation between the two groups with a 25 per cent to 40 per cent overlap; they admitted that their findings could support the continuum view of affective neurotic disorders although they themselves leaned towards the separatist view. During the construction of a self-report scale to assess anxiety and depression in clinical groups, Snaith, Bridge, and Hamilton found that approximately half of both groups of patients, diagnosed as suffering either from endogenous depression or anxiety state, fell into an intermediate area where anxiety symptoms and depressive symptoms were equally balanced; this large group of patients could best be designated by the term 'anxiety-depression'. Downing and Rickels (1974) deprecated the use of such a 'hybrid term' but none the less, in an inquiry based upon self-report, they found that there was a considerable admixture of anxiety and depressive symptoms in their patients.

Outcome studies

Walker (1959) investigated the outcome of 111 patients presenting with affective illness dominated by anxiety symptoms over a period of up to two years; all patients had received the same 'expectant' and supportive treatment with small doses of barbiturate sedatives. One large group in this sample had suffered from a sudden onset of anxiety without major precipitant stress and the prognosis for this group was very much better than for the rest; Walker regarded this form of anxiety state as being basically depressive in nature.

In the third and fourth papers presented by Roth and his colleagues in 1972 (Kerr *et al.*, 1972; Schapira *et al.*, 1972) the outcome of the patients previously diagnosed as suffering from anxiety state or depressive illness was studied. In the fourth paper a follow-up assessment was made by interviewers who were not aware of the original diagnostic assignment of the patients. Whilst symptoms of anxiety and depression had been present in both groups at the time of the original assessment the two groups were distinguished at follow-up by the greater persistence of anxiety-based symptomatology and the overall poorer outcome in the group originally diagnosed as anxiety state. No details were given of the treatment which the patients had received during the key illness and throughout the follow-up period; this was an important omission which was recognized by the authors but discounted as probably irrelevant to their conclusion. However there are dangers in drawing such a conclusion from this type of study. If patients suffering from an arthritic condition, characterized by the symptoms of pain and stiffness, were divided into two groups: those with more pain than stiffness and those with more stiffness than pain, and if the first group were then given a treatment highly effective for pain but only moderately effective for stiffness, while the second group were given a treatment largely ineffective for the relief of both symptoms, then it could be predicted that the outcome of the second group would be poorer than that of the first group; however the statistical confirmation of this prediction would not indicate that the arthritic condition really consisted of two separate entities.

In a follow-up study of 112 patients who had been diagnosed as anxiety neurosis, Clancy, Noyes, Hoenk, and Slymen (1978) found that 44 per cent subsequently suffered from depressive episodes.

Treatment studies

Klein (1964) distinguished two separate types of anxiety according to the response to drugs; he noted that the clinical features of one group were those of sudden onset, hot and cold flashes, panic attacks, palpitations, and a foreboding of death. In a series of such patients he found that 50 per cent had experienced their first panic attack after a threatened or actual separation from a valued person, or bereavement by death, and they were particularly likely to have experienced separation anxiety during their childhood. These patients were shown to respond significantly better to imipramine.

Klein's patients clearly have a close clinical similarity to the patients described by Roth (1959) as suffering from acute anxiety states following calamitous events; such patients were shown by King (1962) to respond to the 'antidepressant' drug phenelzine. It may therefore be that treatment response will serve to redefine clinical categories, at least in the area of affective disorder, but at present the observation that some types of anxiety state respond well to certain drugs conventionally described as antidepressants causes some confusion. In noting the response of phobic anxiety patients to phenelzine (an antidepressant drug of the monoamine oxidase inhibitor group), Tyrer, Candy, and Kelly (1973b) considered the following possibilities: (a) phenelzine is an antidepressant and phenelzine-responsive patients suffer from a depressive illness, entailing considering phobic symptoms as depressive equivalents; (b) phenelzine is an anxiolytic and phenelzine-responsive patients are primarily anxious. There is of course a further possibility not considered above and this is that both depressive and anxiety symptoms may be manifestations of the same core affective illness and that phenelzine is an 'anti-affective' drug rather than being antidepressant or anxiolytic in a narrow sense.

Mendels, Weinstein, and Cochrane (1972), in a study of the relationship between anxiety and depression, considered the following possibilities:

1. It may be that anxiety and depressive states have different biological substrates but that much of the symptomatology of the conditions is similar.

2. That the two conditions represent the same reaction to external or internal stress but the characteristic symptomatology is a reflection of the personality structure of the individual.

3. Anxiety and depressive states originally have different symptoms but, as the severity of the condition increases, secondary symptoms of the other type of disorder make their appearance; in other words chronically anxious patients become depressed and chronically depressed patients develop anxiety. Hays (1964) showed that neurotic symptoms, such as anxiety, may precede the development of the full clinical picture of a psychotic depressive illness and such symptoms, acquired during such an illness, may persist for a long period after recovery from the major depressive manifestation.

At present the matter of the categorical or dimensional hypothesis of the classification of affective disorder has not been settled and will remain unresolved until greater attention is paid to the definition of clinical samples; for both depressive states and anxiety neurosis are broad descriptive terms which cover heterogeneous groups of disorders. In defining clinical samples the matter of age must in future receive greater attention (Pollitt and Young, 1971).

THE PHOBIC NEUROSES

The background to present concepts of phobias

The term phobia is derived from the Greek word *phobos*, meaning fear or terror. Since antiquity there have been descriptions of individuals who suffered from a morbid degree of fear of circumstances which would not be expected to call forth such perturbation. Robert Burton, in his *Anatomy of melancholy* gave examples of several famous people who were afflicted, including Augustus Caesar who dared not sit alone in the dark, and he wrote of Montanus who:

> . . . speaks of one who durst not walk alone from home for fear that he may swoon or die. . . . Another dare not go over a bridge, come near a pool, rock, steep hill, lie in a chamber where cross beams are, for fear he may be tempted to hang, drown or precipitate himself.

Errera (1962) traced the historical evolution of the concept of phobias, which included the medical writings of the 18th and 19th centuries; probably the most influential of these was that of the German neurologist Westphal, for in his monograph *Die Agoraphobie*, written in 1872, he introduced a psychopathological term which is still in current use today. The careful description of three male patients is worth noting:

> . . . impossibility of walking through certain streets or squares, or the possibility of doing so only with resulting dread of anxiety . . . no loss of consciousness . . . no hallucinations or delusions to cause this strange fear . . . agony was much increased at those hours when the particular streets were deserted and the shops closed. The patients derived great comfort from the companionship of men or even an inanimate object such as a vehicle or cane. The use of beer or wine also allowed the patient to pass through the feared locality with comparative comfort. One man even sought, without immoral motives, the companionship of a prostitute as far as his own door . . . Case 3 also had a dislike for crossing a certain bridge . . . there was also apprehension of impending insanity.

The last sentence indicates that, in at least one of the patients, there was a marked degree of generalized anxiety, probably panic attacks, as well as the specific fear of certain localities. Two years earlier Benedikt had used the term *Platzchwindel* (dizziness in public places) for the same syndrome and this term emphasized the somatic manifestations of anxiety; however, it was Westphal's term, agoraphobia, which was adopted by psychiatrists and led to the classification of these locomotor anxieties alongside other conditions of morbid fear, such as the zoöphobias, in which there is little generalized anxiety.

Freud's view of the nature of phobias underwent marked transformation during the course of his writings and these have been summarized by the editors of *The standard edition of the complete psychological works* (Volume 3, p. 83). In the paper on *Obsessions and phobias* Freud (1895) divided the group of phobias into two classes, common and contingent phobias. Common phobias were exaggerated fears of things which are, to some extent, feared by everyone such as solitude, death, the dark, and snakes; contingent phobias were fears of special conditions which inspire no fear in the normal man and among these he included 'agoraphobia and other phobias of locomotion' which he considered to be a simple manifestation of an anxiety neurosis. Since at that time he held a physiological view of anxiety and considered it to be due to 'accumulated sexual tension produced by abstinence or by unconsummated sexual excitation' he believed that phobias, and especially agoraphobia, should be distinguished from hysteria and obsessions which were psychoneuroses and had their origins in the suppression of unacceptable ideas:

> The mechanism of phobias is entirely different from that of obsessions. Substitution is no longer the predominant feature in the former; psychological analysis reveals no incompatible, replaced idea in them. Nothing is ever found but the emotional state of anxiety, which, by a kind of selective process, brings up all the ideas adapted to become the subject of a phobia. In the case of agoraphobia etc., we often find the recollection of the anxiety attack and what the patient really fears is the occurrence of such an attack under the special conditions in which he believes he cannot escape it.

For a period of fifteen years Freud made little further reference to phobias, perhaps because he was perplexed by his own phobias of death and of travelling (*Todesangst* and *Reisefieber*) which, according to his biographer Ernest Jones (1964), afflicted him at that time and appeared to have their roots in alternating mood swings of elation and depression. However, by 1909, with the publication of the case of *Little Hans*, he considered that at least one type of phobia resembled hysteria and was therefore susceptible to psychological analysis; for this he introduced the term anxiety hysteria. By 1933 Freud had developed the 'displacement' view of the nature of phobias; in the lecture *Anxiety and instinctual life* he stated:

> In phobias it is very easy to observe the way in which this internal danger is transformed into an external one—that is to say, how a neurotic anxiety is changed into an apparently realistic one. In order to simplify what is often a very complicated business, let us suppose that the agoraphobic patient is invariably afraid of feelings of temptation that are aroused in him by meeting people in the street. In his phobia he brings about a displacement and henceforward is afraid of an external situation. What he gains by this is obviously that he thinks he will be able to protect himself better that way. One can save oneself from an external danger by flight; fleeing from an internal danger is a difficult enterprise.

In the wake of Freudian psychoanalysis there occurred a diversity of symbolic interpretations of phobias; a brief survey of the literature (Snaith, 1968) revealed the following list of supposed factors underlying the psychogenesis of agoraphobia:

1. Anxiety in the street represents unconscious temptation: the idea of the open street is conceived as an opportunity for sexual adventures; the idea of being alone as a temptation to masturbate.

2. The feared street is conceived of as a place where one might be seen and caught; being alone means being unprotected against the punishing power of the bogeyman.

3. Fear of the street is a defence against exhibitionism and scoptophilia.

4. 'The street can assume various symbolic meanings, which will change according to the phase of the analysis. Thus the street and bridge would symbolize the penis at one stage of the treatment . . . and at a later stage would mean the bedroom, and the street traffic parental intercourse' (Katan, 1951).

This last example might appear a little less fanciful if it is recalled that the word *Verkehr*, in the German language, is used in the context of both street traffic and 'sexual traffic' i.e. sexual intercourse. At any rate it is clear that psychiatrists were being increasingly influenced by the idea that neurotic behaviour developed in an attempt to ward off unacceptable impulses, a defence mechanism which was to become known as reaction-formation.

The concept of phobias as learned symptoms

For it is certain that there is an affinity between the motions of the mother and the child in her womb, so that whatsoever is displeasing to the one offends the other; and the smell of roses may have caused some great headache in the child when it was in its cradle; or a cat may have affrighted it, and none took note of it, nor the child so much as remembered it though the idea of that aversion he then had to roses or a cat remained imprinted in his brain to his life's end (quoted by Errera, 1962).

So wrote Descartes in the middle of the 17th century and just as it is certain that Sigmund Freud was not the first to conceive of the idea of repressed ideas causing symptoms, so the land of thought now claimed by behaviourism has had its shores sighted before in the history of ideas. One of the early and seminal experiments was reported by Watson and Rayner in 1920 and the subject, Albert, became as famous in the annals of behaviourism as did his contemporary in another continent, Little Hans in Freudian psychodynamic theory. Albert was apparently a rather fearless infant; at any rate, he was not afraid of white rats so the experimenters planned to make him so. Accordingly, they clanged an iron bar just behind the child's head on two occasions when the child reached out to touch the rat; a week later, five further paired presentations of the rat and the noise were made and on the eighth trial, when the rat alone was put before Albert, he crawled rapidly away; moreover, the fear response persisted and was reported to have undergone stimulus generalization to all white furry objects including the white beard on a Santa Claus mask. As a basis for further experiment and as a clue to understanding the genesis of phobias, the experiment had an important role but perhaps Watson (1930) had taken too bold a leap from the psychology laboratory to the complexities of psychopathology when he wrote, in connection with the Albert experiment: 'There is thus a thoroughly sound way of accounting for transferred emotional responses – and for the Freudian's "free-floating" affects.' At this time also Mary Cover Jones (1924) was studying children's fears in an institution for the temporary care of children; the fear reactions reported were generally to small animals, rabbits, frogs, and so on because these were kept as pets in the institution and so were available for study. In her brief report Jones stated that verbal appeal, elimination through disuse, negative adaptation, 'repression', and 'distraction' were all observed to be ineffective in eliminating the fear response; 'disuse' referred to the non-appearance of the fear stimulus for a period of some weeks, 'negative adaptation' was the term used for continued contact with the feared stimulus, 'repression' meant shaming the child out of his fear, and 'distraction' referred to the presence of some object of interest to the child alongside the feared object. Two methods were reported to be more successful in leading to an elimination of the fears: direct conditioning and social imitation. In the first of these the feared stimulus was introduced at a time when the child was experiencing pleasure through the satisfaction of hunger and 'social imitation' was the method of overcoming fear by observing other children experiencing pleasure from contact with the object e.g. playing with the rabbit. All these examples were reported briefly and without much conviction but the work was encouraged by Watson himself and was accepted into the growing literature on behaviourism.

Many experiments have shown that fear responses can be produced by conditioning techniques. Miller (1948) showed that fear itself could act as a drive for further learning and, working with rats, he demonstrated that escape from fear (drive reduction) served to reinforce learning. Symptomatic behaviour, especially phobias, came to be viewed as a learned response to aversive stimuli but although the Albert paradigm could be held to be true for a great number of fear responses in animals and normal children and adults it was possibly misleading when directly translated into the more complex field of psychopathology. Olley and McAllister (1974) have shown that there are profound differences between student volunteers with phobias and phobic patients in a clinic sample as regards neuroticism, anxiety, and general psychiatric symptomatology in spite of the two groups sharing a common disabling symptom; the authors conclude that their findings must cast some doubt on the validity of studies on volunteers as analogues of treatment in the clinic setting.

Wolpe (1958), in his classic work *Psychotherapy by reciprocal inhibition*, introduced the concept that, if a response incompatible with anxiety was introduced whilst the patient was exposed to the source of his anxiety then, on repeated performance, the fear would be gradually extinguished. On this principle he developed the therapeutic procedure which he called systematic desensitization and thereby added a powerful boost to the development of behavioural methods of treatment of the neuroses. Neurosis was defined as 'any persistent habit of unadaptive behaviour acquired by learning in a physiologically normal organism'. Although he recognized that neuroses were acquired in anxiety-generating situations he attempted to reduce most of the elements of the disorders to the stimulus-response model of learning theory; to quote from a later paper (1964):

> There are some psychiatrists who say that while they can understand how anxiety reactions triggered by specific stimuli may be subject to deconditioning, they do not see how conditioning can be relevant to anxiety that is present all the time and in all situations. They suggest that there is a variety of neurotic anxiety that has no stimulus antecedents. . . . But if neuroses are due to learning, continuous anxiety that is actually neurotic must also be due to learning. Observations on patients reveal three conditioned sources of continuous anxiety.
>
> 1. The patient may be continuously anxious in all situations except when a specific 'security-object' is present. For example there are cases of agoraphobia in which the patient is free from anxiety only when an intimate person is near him.

2. There may be a conditioned habit of dwelling upon contents of thought that would evoke anxiety in almost everybody. One finds most often, continual imaginings of scenes of the patients death or that of loved ones.

3. There may be true 'free-floating anxiety', which I have suggested be renamed pervasive anxiety. This anxiety is not attributable to any clear-cut stimulus configuration either in thought or the outer world, but appears to be conditioned to various more or less pervasive aspects of stimulation in general. The most pervasive aspects of experience are the awareness of space, time and one's own body (Kant, 1781). Any or all of these may be conditioned to anxiety. Less pervasive concomitants of experience such as light-and-shade contrasts may also be conditioned. . . . A fourth kind of continuous anxiety is not due to conditioning but occurs with exposure to an ongoing conflict situation, such as an undesired marriage. Here we have unconditioned anxiety, that is automatically generated when the organism has simultaneous impulses to opposing actions.

This attempt to interpret continuous anxiety in terms of conditioned reflexes has a certain Procrustean quality. The first source Wolpe cited is not a cause of anxiety but a description of a state which is relieved by a certain condition; the second, the continual brooding on death and disaster is surely not the cause but rather the result of the patient's experience of continuous anxiety, and the third source carries no satisfactory explanation as to why only some people should develop conditioned anxiety to such pervasive features of their environment. It is, in fact, only the fourth source that is acceptable as a *cause* of anxiety and this, Wolpe admits, is *unconditioned* anxiety.

Other authors, such as Dollard and Miller (1950) and, more recently, Stampfl and Levis (1968), have taken a broader view of learning mechanisms in the genesis of clinical neuroses and, in various ways, have attempted an integration with other aetiological factors. Lief (1955) is one of the few authors specifically to analyse phobias from a dualistic approach. He was concerned with the sensory associations in the selection of phobias and regarded the situation at the time of the critical attack of anxiety as being the major determinant in the 'selection' of the phobic object, but the anxiety itself is likely to have other origins. The view of authors such as Lief offers a better understanding and application of knowledge about conditioning to the majority of phobias seen in clinical practice for most of these neuroses, even those relatively specific ones commencing in later life, are found to have their origin at a time when the patient was in an abnormal mood state; whether the disordered mood resulted from conflict or loss or was better understood as an endogenous process, an attack of anxiety in proximity to say a cat, or a visit to a supermarket initiates the phobic neurosis which may persist as an avoidance response long after the resolution of the original mood disorder.

Definition, epidemiology, and classification of phobias

Marked fears of certain objects and situations such as thunderstorms, lifts, and cats are widespread in the population and there is no clear dividing line between a strong fear of a situation and a phobia. Marks (1969) in his book *Fears and phobias* has defined a phobia on four criteria:

1. Fear is out of proportion to the demands of the situation;
2. It cannot be explained or reasoned away;
3. It is beyond voluntary control;
4. The fear leads to an avoidance of the feared situation.

The last of these criteria is not absolute or necessary to the definition for the degree of avoidance will depend upon numerous personal factors and the demands for non-avoidance; it is possible for a person to have a true phobia of air travel and yet to use such transport, albeit with great discomfort, since his business activity depends upon him doing so. A fifth criterion might be added to the above list, which is that a phobia produces some degree of suffering and/or impediment to leading life to the full; this leaves in question whether a city dweller in Britain, with a strong fear of snakes, may ever be said to suffer from a phobia since he can lead life to the full without ever coming into contact with snakes and therefore his fear causes no suffering or handicap apart from inability to visit zoos and to watch nature films.

The most informative survey of the prevalence of phobias was carried out by Agras, Sylvester, and Oliveau (1969) in an area which they considered to be representative of smaller cities in the United States. Trained interviewers contacted 325 people (94 per cent of a sample); the interview was based upon items in a fear questionnaire supplemented by information concerning the duration and intensity of fear and avoidance behaviour and attempts at treatment by family members, clergy, physicians, and others. The degree of fear reported for each item was graded as mild, severe, or of phobic intensity and all respondents who reported phobias were interviewed by psychiatrists. The total prevalence of phobias was estimated to be 76·9/1000 and of these 2·2/1000 were considered to be severely disabling; criteria for determination of the latter degree of severity were perhaps unduly strict for they consisted of absence from work or inability to manage common household tasks. The most common phobias were of illness or injury, followed by storms, various animal phobias, and agoraphobia in that order; most of the phobias were commoner in women than in men but a finding of considerable interest was that fears of the agoraphobic variety were of equal prevalence between the sexes. Whereas the prevalence of certain fears such as snakes and injections showed a peak in the period of adolescence and a decline with age thereafter, other fears, such as crowds, showed a gradually rising prevalence with a peak in late middle age; although the authors do not report upon it, it is probable that agoraphobia belongs to the latter group which leads to a supposition that fears of this sort may be linked to some forms of affective illness, the prevalence of which also rises in middle age. A further finding of importance was that agoraphobia, unlike other fears, is very rarely reported except at phobic intensity and this suggests that agoraphobia has a special psychopathological quality which distinguishes it from other types of phobia.

A five-year follow-up study was carried out on the people identified as having phobias in this survey (Agras, Chapin, and Oliveau 1972). It was found that in children and adolescents phobias improved without specific treatment whereas more long-standing phobias in adults naturally have a poorer prognosis.

An age-of-onset study in a clinical population was carried out by Marks and Gelder (1966). They found that patients suffering from specific animal phobias had a mean age of onset of four years whereas the mean age of onset of other specific phobias (e.g. heights, darkness, thunderstorms) was 23 years, of social phobias 19 years, and of agoraphobia 24 years; they concluded that animal phobias may have a different psychopathological basis to the other groups of phobias and they supported this conclusion by the finding that the former had more circumscribed phobias and a better response to behaviour therapy despite the more prolonged course of the neurosis.

Marks (1969) subdivided the phobic neuroses as follows:

1. Phobias of external stimuli
   a. Agoraphobia
   b. Social phobias
   c. Animal phobias
   d. Miscellaneous specific phobias

2. Phobias of internal stimuli
   e. Illness phobias
   f. Obsessive phobias.

This classification has the merits of being based upon observations of the age of onset, of the degree of associated psychiatric disturbance, of the prognosis, of certain physiological characteristics, and on the response to treatment by behaviour therapy. There are however, some difficulties with such a scheme which must now be considered.

Agoraphobia

This term is a misleading diagnostic label for a group of conditions which are not homogeneous and have in common only a certain type of feared situation. Etymologically the term means a fear of gatherings of people in the open, for the Greek *agora* means market-place, which in the warm climate of the country was held in the open; however, the term is usually applied when the patient has at least one or more fears among the following constellation: leaving home or other shelter, congregations of people whether in the open or in closed buildings, wide open spaces, narrow confined spaces and streets, being alone, and travelling. In addition to the central fears it is usually assumed that the patient will manifest a high level of general anxiety and may experience panic attacks, pervasive fear, and apprehensive dread of some undefined calamity, somatic symptoms of anxiety, and sometimes depersonalization. In addition there may be a diffuse collection of other phobias which frequently include situations of potential threat such as hospitals and witnessing violent behaviour. The central constellation of fears are certainly of diverse origin. Buglass *et al.* (1977) identified a fear of becoming ill, often accompanied by a fear of causing a public disturbance, as being central to the agoraphobic complex. However, an examination of a large series of patients identified as suffering from agoraphobia would distinguish two main types of unrelated fears; there are those with illness fears that they may swoon or die and no one be near to help them and these patients, like Westphal's patients have a dread of deserted places; the other group have a fear of being under public scrutiny and for this reason avoid crowded places but feel more comfortable in deserted places. These patients have a strong resemblance to certain types of phobic patients with social phobias. In some patients the degree of free-floating anxiety may be very severe, in others it may be moderate and in yet others it may be absent and in this latter group the 'agoraphobia' may have the characteristics of a monosymptomatic phobic neurosis. In other patients, depression rather than anxiety is the main pattern of emotional disorder; in the depressed patients the agoraphobia, on closer analysis, is based upon a marked reluctance, rather than fear, of going out of the home and the probability of meeting an acquaintance with the consequent required effort to appear cheerful or interested in the latest gossip.

It is therefore clear that patients may be classified under the label of agoraphobia who in fact suffer from a range of disorders—from the overwhelming anxiety of Roth's calamity syndrome, through frankly depressive states, multiple phobias with little other psychiatric disturbance, down to single fears of fairly circumscribed situations. It may be argued that if a large group of 'agoraphobics' are studied then it will be found that their course, age of onset, or the presence of other symptoms distinguishes them from some other class such as patients with animal phobias; however such findings merely camouflage the fact that 'agoraphobia' is in fact a heterogeneous collection of disorders and not a homogeneous entity. As Shafer (1975) put it: 'the syndrome of agoraphobia is multi-faceted and represents, in some, the aftermath of a depressive illness frequently still unresolved when treatment for the phobia is requested. In others it consists of maladaptive conditioned responses maintained by habit, while still other sufferers are prone to a variety of psychological conflicts and primary or secondary gains that play an integral part in the formation and maintenance of phobic symptoms.'

Social phobia

The grounds for considering phobias concerned with interpersonal situations to be a distinct psychopathological entity is also dubious and is probably based upon the finding that any large group of patients with such phobias will be found to suffer from a degree of generalized anxiety intermediate to the groups conventionally classed as agoraphobia and those with specific phobias. Many, but by no means all patients with social phobias experience a marked degree of somatized anxiety in their feared situation, such as blushing, tremor of the hands, or choking on food. Sometimes patients who develop such phobias have no abnormality of personality structure and first develop the phobia in the setting of a traumatic situation such as vomiting in the midst of a crowd at a party; the phobia may have its origin in a state of depression or generalized anxiety, which may have resolved, leaving the phobia as a permanent aftermath of the affective disorder. Others may develop the phobia on the basis of a particular type of personality structure characterized by generalized social insecurity and sensitivity to criticism, real or imagined, by others; in the setting of such a personality background, some relatively minor stress such as a difficult interview with someone in authority, being caught out in the act of some deception, or even being praised for some achievement, may be sufficient to precipitate a phobia.

Social phobia, therefore, like agoraphobia, is not a homogeneous clinical entity but represents the prominent symptomatic manifestation of a wide variety of psychological disorders and psychiatric illnesses. Sometimes, as already mentioned, the distinction between agoraphobia and social phobia may be confused. Kraüpl Taylor (1966), for instance, refers to some women with such severe degrees of fear of being looked at by others that they are only able to leave the house when it is dark or foggy. One may speculate that the 'agoraphobic' who habitually wears dark glasses is really a 'social phobic' in disguise.

Specific phobias

The finding of Marks and Gelder that adult patients with specific phobias of animate objects had a younger age of onset than those with specific phobias of other objects or situations is an interesting observation but may be hard to replicate. Many patients with animal phobias do in fact have a later age of onset of their neurosis and many patients with fears of hospitals, hypodermic injections, thunderstorms, and being alone in the dark, trace the origin of their phobia back to infancy.

The number and variety of objects and situations which may become associated with morbid fear of phobic intensity is practically

without limit; some of the more common phobias have been digni-
fied with Greek or Latin prefixes, such as acrophobia (fear of
heights), ailurophobia (cats), astraphobia (lightning), and so on; a
more extended list of these may be seen in Marks's *Fears and phobias*;
however if it were necessary for such a term to be applied to every
specific phobia seen by psychiatrists then a scholar of classical
languages would be kept in full-time employment for that purpose
alone; two recent examples in the author's clinic were a phobia of
breaking wind in public and a phobia of the sound of cutlery
striking against crockery.

Specific phobias are seldom so specific as the apellation may
signify; there is often a generalization of fear to similar or related
objects so that the patient with a phobia of cats also dislikes the
touch of all furry objects. Moreover, the phobia with which a person
presents has often assumed such overwhelming proportions that he
overlooks and fails to mention other phobias which are frequently
only elicited when he completes a checklist of common phobias.
Likewise, other lesser degrees of neurotic disability are frequently
overlooked by both the patient and the psychiatrist unless specific
inquiry is made; for example a patient was successfully treated for
what appeared to be an isolated phobia of crane flies ('Daddy long-
legs'); at the conclusion of her treatment she expressed her relief that
a mild obsessional checking ritual had also cleared up although this
had not been previously mentioned during either the examination or
at any stage in the treatment. More obvious mood disturbance is
clearly evident in many patients who, in addition to their distressing
phobia, suffer from generalized states of anxiety or depression;
sometimes the mood disorder may be considered to be secondary to
the long-standing phobic neurosis but this is not always so certain
and some patients with severe phobias are relieved of their fear when
a mild and sometimes overlooked depressive state is successfully
treated.

School phobia

School phobia (or, as some authors prefer to call it, school refusal)
is, like agoraphobia in older people, not a homogeneous disorder;
although the defining symptom, a fear of school, may lend a sem-
blance of uniformity, none the less children with this symptom show
a varied clinical picture of diverse aetiology. The use of the label
school phobia also tends to mask the fact that the disorder has no

distinct boundary but shades off into other neurotic disorders in which the child may have no fear of school but experiences abdominal pains on Monday mornings or feels faint in the morning school assembly. There is no uniform age at which the condition manifests itself and it may first occur during attendance at the child's first school or be delayed until adolescence. Onset may be sudden or gradual and may or may not coincide with a particular upset in the child's home or a specific psychotraumatic incident at school. There is no single attitude towards school and many children who develop the condition have shown good progress with no previous difficulty in any specific aspect of school life and work. Neither is the home background of the child or his relationship with his parents marked by any constant pattern although most authors have noted that neurotic disorder and a history of psychiatric treatment in the parents is common. It is probable that the majority of children who develop the symptom have some dependency problems before their school phobia becomes manifest. The child with a 'typical' school phobia will experience severe anxiety centred around attempts to go to school and many will be quite unable to enter the school premises voluntarily; there will normally be a marked somatization of anxiety, often abdominal pains and sickness or diarrhoea occurring before the hours of school attendance. When at home the child does not appear to be severely anxious but an account will be given that there has been some change in mood so that he appears moody or irritable; there are not any other specific neurotic symptoms and the child can leave the home and be separated from his mother on some errand, such as a trip to the local shop, without displaying anxiety or concern. The child, his parents, and his teachers are all unable to give any satisfactory explanation for such a dramatic and distressing change of behaviour although some reasons may be found to justify it.

It is stressed that such a description as this so-called 'typical' presentation of the condition is given only in order that the varieties of the disorder may be considered. Two examples will clarify the varieties of clinical picture which may be subsumed under the label of 'school phobia'.

> John was a timid, unassertive youth aged 11 who stammered slightly when speaking to strangers; at his first school he had made one friend, but he rarely joined in school activities or left the home in the evenings or during school holidays and never went to parties in the homes of other

children; his chief interest was in his pet animals. He made a poor relationship with his parents who, being involved in their own relationship difficulties, tended to show little interest in him and rarely encouraged him. His elder brother ignored him except on the rare occasions when he made some disparaging remark. When John moved to the middle school he lost his only friend and felt lonely in the new school environment; one of the teachers seemed to dislike him and found frequent opportunity to criticize his poor work performance; other children found his unassertiveness an easy target for bullying and stupid pranks and he earned a shameful nickname. He became depressed and increasingly unwilling to go to school. His parents showed no understanding of his difficulties and threatened all kinds of impractical punishments which only increased John's demoralization and strengthened him in a mulish refusal to attend school.

Jane was the only child of her parents. Her mother suffered from an anxiety state in which fear of being on her own was a prominent symptom; the father was a merchant seaman. When Jane was approaching school age her mother's anxiety state worsened and when school started she was kept at home on the slightest pretext. After she had been at school for about a year her mother took an overdose of tablets leaving a written note that Jane should be looked after by an aunt. The mother then spent two months in a psychiatric hospital and Jane was not taken to see her; the child became frightened, thinking her mother had died and that no one would tell her. She continued going to school but when the mother returned home she became increasingly anxious about separation and on several occasions ran home from school to see if her mother was all right. The mutual anxiety of mother and daughter increased and finally Jane developed night terrors, and a multitude of somatic symptoms and refused to go to school or to be out of sight of her mother for more than a few minutes.

These examples, together with the vignette of the 'typical' case give some idea of the complexity of factors that may result in the neurotic symptom of school phobia. In many cases a variety of personality disorders, relationship problems, neurosis in the parents, and specific problems at school are found in varying proportions. The association between school phobia in children and neurotic disorder in the parents has been studied by Berg, Butler, and Pritchard (1974) who found that about 20 per cent of mothers of school phobic adolescents suffered from psychiatric disorder and of these about half suffered from an affective disorder. Tyrer and Tyrer (1974) interviewed 60 phobic, 60 anxious, and 60 neurotic depressed adults and compared their samples with a control group. Their findings suggested a link between school refusal and adult neurotic disorder and, by implication, between childhood and adult neurosis although there was rarely a continuous development of the neurotic condition; more commonly an intervening period of improved mental health was recorded. Berg, Butler, and Hall (1976) followed up 100 school phobic adolescents three years after discharge from an in-patient psychiatric unit (the fact that they were in-patients indicated that they had suffered from the more severe forms of the disorder); they observed that severe school phobia in early adolescence resembled adult affective disorders in some clinical features and in outcome. Hersov (1977) surveyed the syndrome of school phobia and commented upon the relationship between the symptom and underlying affective disorder. The evidence certainly points to a strong probability that a proportion of the children suffer from an affective disorder. If this is the case then it is probable that these children will present with the more 'typical' features described above, in which symptoms arise, unlike as in John and Jane, for little understandable reason. The presentation of a mood disorder of irritability and anxiety, rather than depression, is in keeping with the age-dependence of these symptoms within the spectrum of affective disorder and the finding that a proportion of school phobic children respond favourably to antidepressant drug treatment (Frommer, 1968; Gittleman-Klein and Klein, 1971) lends further support to this thesis.

The aetiology of phobic neuroses

Many factors contribute to the genesis of a phobic neurosis. Among these are the constitutional liability of the individual to develop prolonged fear reactions, the personality structure, the selection and successful employment of coping mechanisms in the early stages of the neurosis, the attitudes of family, friends and professional advisers, the potential threat, real or symbolic, of any original psycho-traumatic event, the presence of a mood disorder at the onset of the neurosis and its persistence or recurrence, and finally the presence and degree of secondary gain from the neurosis.

Personality structure
It is probable that some degree of abnormality of a specific personality trait underlies the liability to develop a phobic neurosis although this has not been defined nor is it apparently universally present. All

investigations of the supposed premorbid personality structure of phobic patients or any other group of neurotics are befogged by the frequently insurmountable difficulties of determining just when the neurotic disorder commenced and whether supposed abnormalities of the personality were not highly coloured by a neurotic state which may have been present for a long time but in milder degree. Difficulties of this kind are particularly intractable in the case of the agoraphobic syndrome, in which mild episodes of anxiety neurosis may have preceded the appearance of the recognized phobic state over a prolonged period of time (Snaith, 1968; Mendel and Klein, 1969). The occurrence of such neurotic episodes in the past will probably have resulted in states of dependency, hostility, sensitivity, hopelessness, and all kinds of emotional turmoil which are sometimes judged to be part of the basic personality of all agoraphobic patients. An example is provided by Terhune (1949) who considered that agoraphobic patients were: 'constitutionally unusually suggestible, imaginative and sensitive, with considerable drive, high standards of conduct and exceedingly active intelligence and ambition, and were reared "soft" but usually by neurotic parents on one of whom they are still emotionally dependent'; however, he remarked that these patients had suffered from a number of childhood phobias and one can only speculate whether the supposedly universal characteristic of dependency was really basic to the personality structure or resulted from early experience of neurotic symptoms and the method of management of these by parents. Roth (1959) published a careful description of patients suffering from the phobic-anxiety depersonalization syndrome; on the whole they were assessed as being more dependent, immature, obsessional and anxiety-prone, and more afflicted with chronic but mild phobias than other neurotic patients; the relationship of the female patients with their mothers was described as intense, excluding contact with others in the family circle and a high proportion were sexually frigid before the onset of the severe neurosis. However, this general picture was subject to conspicuous exceptions, and examples were cited of patients who had previously faced and successfully surmounted responsibilities and stress for years before the breakdown occurred. Marks and Gelder (1965) remarked upon the premorbid personality of a group of 21 patients with travel phobias (agoraphobia) and a group of 11 with mixed specific and social phobias; the former had suffered from a greater variety of neurotic symptoms and over half of them had neurotic traits in childhood. However, for neither the agoraphobic group nor the group with other phobias, could any typical personality structure be detected.

All that can be said with any degree of certainty about patients suffering from phobic neurosis is that, by the nature of their disorder, they show some degree of dependency on others and that the more generalized the neurotic disturbance the more likely is dependency to be pronounced. Many adult patients who manifest phobic symptoms in the setting of a general mood disturbance are likely to have suffered from phobic problems in childhood and it is probable that the majority of patients who develop social phobias do so in the setting of some degree of personal sensitivity to the opinions of others. More exact information is unlikely to result from retrospective personality assessments of patients who present with phobic neuroses but may be provided by long-term prospective studies in which large numbers of young children are followed through to adult life.

Attitudes of the individual and the reaction of others

The outcome of a fear, and whether it becomes more intense and hardens into a phobic neurosis, will depend to a large extent on the attitudes of the individual and the reaction of others to his fear. Some examples will make this clear.

> A child developed a fear of worms after another child playfully slipped one into his strawberries and cream; the mother was horrified by the incident and forbade the playmate to come to the home again. Thus for the child a trivial incident developed into a shameful act which was of sufficient gravity to lead to the loss of a friend. A few days later, when playing in the garden, he trod on a worm, immediately felt frightened and ran into the house; when his mother asked why he was so upset he dared not confess to the shameful contact with the worm, lied to her, and cried himself to sleep. Thereafter he avoided playing in the garden and when, after a further few days, another playmate who had heard of the incident with the strawberries, mockingly threw a worm at him his fear became established as an enduring phobia.

In this case the reaction of the mother was the crucial factor in the genesis of the phobia. To take another example, this time where the attitude of the individual is the more important factor:

> A young woman and her boyfriend were both involved in a car accident, the man being the driver of the vehicle; she had always distrusted his driving ability and was also inclined to distrust him in other matters. He

was dependent on the car for his livelihood and commenced driving again without too much difficulty but she was now sensitized to car journeys and, in spite of his taking rather elaborate care when they were driving together, she remained nervous. A week later a dog rushed at the car and was killed and there followed an angry scene between the dog owner and the young man; this incident promoted the young woman's fear of cars to phobic severity which rapidly generalized to all car transport no matter who was driving.

What Franks (1961) has called the 'assumptive world' of the person is a further factor which is of importance in the genesis of some phobias and other neurotic symptoms. An example of the operation of this factor is the fear of sudden death which develops in some patients who suffer from panic attacks; these sudden, apparently inexplicable, and terrifying episodes are accompanied by palpitations and faintness and a patient who has known some relative or friend die suddenly, is particularly likely to assume that the same fate will shortly overtake himself. In the early stages of the neurosis a careful medical examination, thorough explanation, and calm reassurance will help to reverse this assumption but a contact with a doctor which leaves the patient no wiser will inevitably lead to entrenchment of the phobia. The assumptive world of the individual is again the operative factor in a person who has always assumed that flight is a hazardous undertaking and who develops a phobia of air travel without ever having been in a plane.

The attitude of others, concealed or overt, may sometimes play an important part in the maintenance of a phobic neurosis. This was highlighted by Hafner (1977) who followed up a group of married women who had undergone a programme of treatment for agoraphobia; he found that sometimes the husband's reactions to the prospect of his wife's recovery and his need for her to be ill and dependent on him were so great that recovery was unlikely to take place. Hafner recorded that one husband attempted suicide after his wife's recovery since he felt useless; two men became depressed when the focus of dissatisfaction shifted from the wife's agoraphobia to their own sexual dysfunction and four husbands became abnormally jealous when their wives were able to go out alone, perhaps for the first time in years. As Hafner remarked: 'Any study aimed at understanding phobic disorders in married females which fails to acknowledge the importance of denial in their husbands is unlikely to be fully successful.'

Potential threat and significance of the psychotraumatic incident

The potential threat of a psychotraumatic incident may be an important factor in determining the onset of a phobic neurosis; the threat may be actual or may occur only in fantasy. A building worker may develop a phobia for heights if he loses his foothold a long way from ground and would have fallen to his death had he not managed to regain his balance. A miner may develop a phobia of descent into the earth following a relatively slight underground accident if he was aware of a recent mining disaster, and a child may first develop a fear of hospitals following the sudden departure of his mother to hospital in circumstances of anxiety and pain. A phobia may also develop if the threat occurs only in fantasy; for instance a young woman saw a horror film in which considerable destruction and loss of life resulted from a hurricane; upset and frightened she went to bed, dreamed of storms and death, and awoke to the sound of a high wind and thunderstorm; although she had not previously feared thunderstorms she was terrified by the sound and developed a persisting phobia of storms.

Mood disorder and affective illness

A temporary disturbance of moods may provide the fertile soil in which the seed of a phobic neurosis may first germinate; the phobia may then subside as the mood returns to normal or it may persist as a permanent aftermath of the mood disorder. Many phobic neuroses commence during times of unhappiness, insecurity, or conflict which causes a reactive anxiety or depressive state and, in the setting of this, some trivial incident may be sufficient to cause a prolonged phobia.

> A young mother recently discovered her husband's infidelity and felt her marital security to be threatened; she tried to conceal her feelings of resentment and became depressed. Although she had always been scrupulously honest the thought of stealing a needed article occurred to her whilst shopping in a supermarket; she resisted the sudden temptation but an error occurred at the counter and, when the cashier had to recheck all the articles she had purchased, she felt everyone was looking at her, that they knew about her marital difficulties and suspected her of shoplifting. As soon as she could do so she rushed from the store in a state of panic and was thereafter reluctant to enter any large store or shop; from that time she developed a phobia of stores and was quite unable to enter them.

Patients developing endogenous mood disorder may be at greater risk for the development of phobias since they consider their disturbance of mood to be unexplainable and illogical. If a severe attack of panic occurs in some non-threatening situation the patient comes to associate that situation with his panic and his apprehension concerning approach to the situation leads to further panic and eventually to phobic avoidance. For example, a student, who previously had no academic problems, suffered from an acute depressive illness and experienced an attack of anxiety in a lecture hall; on the next occasion that he attempted to enter the lecture hall he felt anxious, hastily retreated, and the phobia of lecture halls persisted for a long period after he had recovered from the depressive illness.

Several authors have recorded the presence of depressive states preceding or coinciding with the onset of the phobic neurosis. In his retrospective survey of agoraphobic housewives, Roberts (1964) found that 25 per cent had been sufficiently depressed at the onset of the disorder to have received treatment with ECT and this finding leads to the supposition that an even larger proportion of the patients had suffered from milder degrees of depression. Solyom *et al.* (1974) observed that phobic neurosis frequently commenced in the setting of a generalized disturbance of mood, and Jarrett and Schnurr (1979), in a psychometric study of newly admitted psychiatric in-patients, confirmed that diffuse phobias (agoraphobia and social phobias), but not simple phobias, were associated with depression. The most thorough study of the relationship between phobias and affective disorder was carried out by Schapira, Kerr, and Roth (1970) who were engaged in the investigation of a large number of patients who had been admitted to hospital for an anxiety state or a depressive illness. They confirmed that phobias more commonly preceded an anxiety state than a depressive illness and were also more likely to make their first appearance during an anxiety state; however, even in depressive illness, symptoms of the agoraphobic type occurred for the first time in life in 11 per cent and social phobias for the first time in 13 per cent of the sample. The authors made no comment on the liability of phobic symptoms to persist following recovery from the affective disorder but this probably happens in a proportion of patients.

Treatment of anxiety and phobias

The treatment of anxiety-based neuroses must rest upon a careful formulation of the condition of the patient. Many of the conflicting reports of the effectiveness of different therapeutic programmes in these neuroses arises from the definition of the population merely by the categorical label; patients for whom the correct diagnostic assignment is that of either anxiety neurosis or phobic neurosis will not be a homogeneous group of individuals. Even patients within the more restricted subcategory of agoraphobia may be expected to show a considerable variation in response to a specific therapeutic technique if the phobia occurs in the setting of a low-grade depressive state than if it is a relatively encapsulated psychopathological disorder, if it is a chronic disorder than if it is of recent onset, if there is a considerable secondary gain from the neurosis than if the patient's motivation for recovery is strong, and so on. In order to achieve the best results the correct therapeutic technique should be selected after a careful assessment of the following factors:

1. The degree to which the manifest anxiety is a reflection of the basic trait anxiety of the individual or may be considered to be a state arising in the setting of a relatively normal personality structure.

2. The presence, or absence, of stress or conflict which are clearly related, or may reasonably be supposed to be related to the occurrence of the anxiety. Environmental and interpersonal stress is a universal human experience and the anxiety should not automatically be considered to arise from such a factor; an attempt should be made to assess how the patient has coped with similar stress at earlier periods in his life.

3. The present and past life-style of the patient, the range of his interests, activities, and the durability and quality of his relationships with others. These factors will be related to many aspects of the personality structure but of particular importance are those of avoidance of difficulties and dependence on others (Andrews, 1966). The premorbid assessment of these factors will be hard to determine in those patients suffering from long-standing neurotic states.

4. The duration of the neurosis and the past history of fluctuation in severity, remission, and recurrence of symptoms. If periods of improvement or worsening have occurred, an attempt

should be made to determine whether these episodes are related to any particular changes in the circumstances of the patient.

5. The presence of any particular strategies which the patient has developed in order to cope with his symptoms; for instance a woman suffering from social phobias may be attempting to cope with the neurosis by arriving early at social gatherings so that she can obtain a seat near the door. A dangerous coping mechanism is the use of alcohol in order to allay anxiety, for this may lead to alcohol dependence (Mullaney and Trippett, 1979).

6. The attitudes of others towards the patient's neurosis. The comments of Hafner on the attitudes of the spouse of a phobic patient have been noted earlier. An example of a destructive attitude leading to prolongation of the neurosis is that of school phobia in a child whose mother suffers from a fear of being alone and covertly encourages the child's non-attendance at school.

7. Apparent secondary gain from the neurosis; this factor is hard to assess and conclusions should not be reached too readily. The prevalent view that all patients derive some significant gain from their neurosis is untrue. For instance it should not be immediately assumed that a wife who fears to be alone at night is necessarily attempting to derive increased attention from her husband.

8. The presence, or absence, of other psychopathological features. The most important of these are depressive symptoms which may be partly masked by prominent anxiety or phobic symptomatology. The use of an easily completed patient-rated scale such as the irritability-depression-anxiety (IDA) Scale (Snaith *et al.*, 1978) may confirm clinical suspicion of depression and later be used as a measure of severity of the mood states during therapy. Anxiety occurs in the setting of many psychiatric disorders and may, for example, be a prominent symptom of a delirious state or an early symptom of schizophrenia. Diagnostic errors will occur unless the mental state examination is undertaken with care.

9. Response, or non-response, to treatments that have been

used for similar neurotic symptoms in the past. A good referral letter from a general practitioner to a psychiatric department should contain a comprehensive list of any drugs that may have been prescribed, the dosage and the response. Time, and faith, is lost when the psychiatrist, in ignorance of such information, simply repeats procedures which have been proved in the past to be ineffective.

After a formulation of the patient's case the therapeutic approach must be considered but sometimes a delay is advisable; it may be necessary to request to see a relative in order to gain a fuller understanding of the many complex factors that enter into the psychogenesis of all neuroses. A physical examination and sometimes a special investigation (such as an EEG in a suspected temporal lobe epileptic disorder) may be required. Moreover, the exhaustive process of the psychiatric examination may often in itself have a therapeutic effect and the patient may return to a subsequent interview having reevaluated his anxiety in the light of some of the facts about himself and his situation which he has been required to consider during the examination. If a treatment such as a drug (or advice) had been prescribed too hastily at the first interview the improvement may be wrongly attributed to that factor. The first interview should however end with a brief formulation to the patient of the salient points which the clinician has learned during the interview and the patient should be invited to comment upon this formulation and, should he consider it to be necessary, to offer corrections or to add further information about which he has not been asked and which he thinks may be relevant to his case. If the patient has been accompanied by a spouse or close relative he may be asked if he wishes the relative to be present during the formulation; this proposal should not be considered to be obligatory but the very reaction of the patient to the proposal may be informative and, if the relative is seen at this stage, the opportunity is gained for valuable supplemental information concerning the attitude of the relative and the likelihood that his help could usefully be enlisted in the eventual therapeutic programme. Alternatively the impression may be gained that some effort may have to be spent in forthcoming interviews in the attempt to correct antitherapeutic or frankly destructive attitudes. Finally, the patient may be informed that it is understood that morbid anxiety is an extremely uncomfortable state of mind which is frequently alleviated by some understanding of its origin but that, should specific therapy be required, many effective treatments are now available. He should be advised to reflect on the points raised during the formulation before the next interview.

The second interview, which ideally should not be longer than a week since the first, is opened by an inquiry concerning the patient's present mental state and of any change since he was last seen. The provisional formulation, which ended the last interview, should then be reviewed and further additions or corrections requested. If there has been little change in the severity of the anxiety the remainder of the interview should be spent in a consideration of the therapeutic approach. An explanation of what this may entail for the patient together with a brief outline of the rationale of such therapy should be given. Blackwell (1976) is among the many authors who have pointed out that treatment compliance and an ultimately successful outcome of therapy depends to a large degree on the understanding by the patient of what is to be done and why; such an outline is equally valid whether the treatment is to take the form of supportive psychotherapy, some formal psychotherapeutic technique or is to be based largely on drug treatment.

Psychotherapy

Supportive psychotherapy for anxiety-based neuroses should be carried out at weekly sessions each lasting about thirty minutes; more therapeutic time may not be available outside private practice and in fact there is no evidence that the devotion of more time will shorten the recovery process for, as Gelder (1979) has pointed out, the main thrust of the therapeutic effect probably takes place between the sessions with the therapist. During the therapeutic sessions time should be spent in considering the specific cues which elicit anxiety, coping strategies which might be adopted in order to lessen the anxiety whilst at the same time not avoiding it. Readjustment of the life-style and relationships may be necessary if these are clearly pathogenic but the therapist should rarely specifically advise some major change, such as the breaking-off of an engagement or a change of job, but should confine himself to helping the patient to understand how such factors are probably related to the emotional disturbance; the non-directive approach is the important element in Roger's client-centred counselling. Although episodes of morbid anxiety are most uncomfortable and the tendency of the patient is to take measures to avoid them, he will thereby only lead to their perpetuation at the cost of greater personal emotional handicap; an essential element of supportive psychotherapy for anxiety-based neuroses is therefore the encouragement given to the patient to face up to his anxiety and thereby to overcome it. This is the essential curative factor in many psychotherapeutic techniques and was recognized some decades ago by Freud (1917) in the context of psychoanalytic therapy:

> One can hardly ever master a phobia if one waits till the patient lets the analysis influence him to give it up. He will never in that case bring into the analysis the material indispensable for a convincing resolution of the phobia. [With severe agoraphobics] one succeeds only when one can induce them . . . to go into the street and struggle with their anxiety while they make the attempt. One starts therefore by moderating their anxiety so far; and it is only when that has been achieved at the physician's demand that the associations and memories come into the patient's mind which enable the phobia to be resolved.

The great variety of formal psychotherapeutic procedures which are available cannot be considered here, for formal psychotherapeutic techniques may only be described by those with considerable experience of their practice. Therefore, in the present chapter only the techniques subsumed under the term behaviour therapy will be considered whilst a more extended account of a therapeutic approach to anxiety will occur in Chapter 7.

Behavioural psychotherapy

The term behavioural psychotherapy is more appropriate for the employment of behavioural techniques in the clinical setting for it places emphasis on the fact that the techniques are used in the context of the therapeutic relationship and a broader consideration of the circumstances and personal problems of the patient than was originally conceived by the pioneers who introduced the procedures into the corpus of psychiatric treatment. Behaviour therapy was introduced in the belief that it was, in supposed contrast to other psychotherapeutic methods, a 'scientific' method based upon 'modern learning theory' and a list of its distinctive features was compiled in order to establish these claims (Eysenck and Rachman, 1965). Whereas the early theorists tended to ignore the complex nature of neurotic disorders seen in clinical practice and frequently supported their hypotheses by experiments on animals and student volunteers, clinicians soon became aware that, although the techniques were undoubtedly of value, the somewhat mechanistic application of counterconditioning principles did not lead to the best results nor wholly explain the effects.

It was soon realized that the relationship between the therapist and the patient was of importance in determining the outcome of therapy and Meyer and Gelder (1963) considered that it was, in fact, the most important factor. Chesser (1976) has summarized the present concepts involved in the behavioural approach:

> It is wide based, grounded in experimental psychology principles, ready to take cognizance of organismic variables, individual differences, organic pathology, the developmental history of the patient, the factors initiating and maintaining undesired behaviour, the existing behavioural repertoire of the patient (potential assets) and the social environment of the patient.

A gradual rapprochement is taking place between behavioural psychotherapy and other psychotherapeutic approaches. It has been suggested that insight into the psychogenesis of the symptom comes in the wake of successful desensitization and that the success of some psychotherapeutic techniques may be based upon principles to which behaviourists lay claim (Cautela, 1965). After more than two decades, behaviour therapists may be tending to develop an individual therapeutic style which, being based upon optimism and the expectation of early improvement, may contribute markedly towards the overall success rate of the method. In a comment upon the American study comparing behaviour therapy and psychodynamic psychotherapy (Sloane *et al.*, 1975) a leading article in *The Lancet* (1976) stated:

> This study strongly suggested that, despite their mutual antagonism, there is remarkable overlap in the approaches of both groups. Many of the differences seem to be a matter of degree rather than of substance. Behaviour therapists tended to be more directive, more concerned with symptoms, less concerned with childhood memories and, despite their reputation for coldness and lack of clinical involvement, warmer and more active therapists. . . . They made as many interpretive statements as did the psychotherapists. Thus it is not clear whether the two groups, despite their theoretically differing backgrounds, did actually use fundamentally different approaches to reach the same therapeutic end or whether the effectiveness of their treatments was due to factors common

to both schools of thought. The patients themselves seemed in less doubt, and those who improved most attributed their response less to the theoretical framework within which they were treated than to the personality, enthusiasm, and involvement of the individual therapist.

This suggestion that differences in outcome are at least partly due to personal attributes of the therapists, as well as the theoretical structure in which they work, has been pointed out on many occasions but recently most persistently by Truax and his colleagues (e.g. Truax and Mitchell, 1971) who have shown that the qualities of a successful therapist (of whatever persuasion) are, what they term: accurate empathic understanding, non-possessive warmth, and genuineness.

There has been little written on the contribution of behaviour therapy to the management of pervasive anxiety probably because, as stated at the beginning of this chapter, most patients suffering from generalized anxiety states also experience a raising of their anxiety level in certain situations and it is towards this focussed anxiety that behaviour therapists direct their attention. The following discussion will therefore consider the development of behavioural psychotherapy in the management of phobic anxiety.

In the treatment of phobic neuroses Wolpe's technique of systematic desensitization was generally found to be effective in specific phobias but the results in the treatment of the more complex agoraphobic syndrome were held to be disappointing. Systematic desensitization consisted of training the patient in muscular relaxation, construction of a hierarchy of situations eliciting ever greater degrees of anxiety for each patient, and then instructing the patient to envisage the scenes, one at a time, whilst in the relaxed state (Wolpe advised that this should be done while the patient was hypnotized, presumably for the greater clarity of imagery which the patient could thereby achieve); if any scene evoked anxiety this was signalled by the patient, and the next higher scene in the hierarchy was not to be presented until he could persistently tolerate the lower scene without experiencing anxiety. Wolpe stated that one of the reasons for failure of the method lay in the inability of some patients to relax and to obtain a clear image of the scene; it may have been such factors that contributed to the poorer results with agoraphobic patients although many other factors are involved in this syndrome which is much more complex than other phobic neuroses.

The other major behavioural technique for the treatment of

phobias has unfortunately received the rather alarming name of 'flooding' and starts from the premise, opposite to that of systematic desensitization, of encouraging the patient to experience anxiety and to confront his neurotic fears more abruptly. The flooding technique has its origins in three independent sources. Frankl, in Vienna, had introduced a form of psychotherapy based upon existential ideas which he called logotherapy and an element in this method was the technique called paradoxical intention. The technique is described in a short paper (Frankl, 1960); in essence the patient is encouraged to deliberately produce and even exaggerate his neurotic symptoms. Among the examples he gives to illustrate the principle, is that of a young medical student who feared that whilst dissecting at the Institute of Anatomy she would begin to tremble when the anatomy instructor entered the room; having heard Frankl lecture she decided to put his principles into practice and in order to demonstrate to the instructor the enormity of her neurotic symptom she said to herself, every time the instructor entered the room 'Oh here is the instructor! Now I'll show him what a good trembler I am—I'll really show him how I can tremble.' Whenever she deliberately tried to produce the tremor she was unable to do so and she overcame her neurosis. Frankl advised that the instructions on paradoxical intention should be carried out in as humorous a setting as possible but it is obvious that the patient should understand that the technique is a genuine and a successful one and that the therapist is not merely mocking him. Certainly the method can be very successful in a very short time and perhaps is the only technique available when time is limited to a few days; for instance a patient had to make an important business trip by plane which he knew to be impossible on account of his severe flight phobia; he requested to be cured within five days. He was therefore instructed to make a daily trip to the nearest airport and to spend three hours looking at the planes taking off and to imagine himself entering them; he was also instructed to make himself feel as anxious as possible in the process. On the appointed day he undertook the flight in comparative comfort.

An almost identical procedure was reported by a physician to a student health service (Malleson, 1959), who undertook to treat a foreign student for severe examination phobia who presented only a few days before his exam. The student was instructed deliberately to bring on his fear by imagining himself in the exam hall and when he succeeded in doing so it waned in half an hour; he was then instructed not to push his fear aside but every time he experienced a little spasm to augment it deliberately and if he did not spontaneously experience anxiety every 20 or 30 minutes he was to make a special effort to do so. A few days later the student sat his examination without difficulty. Malleson proposed the term 'reactive inhibition therapy' for the technique.

A third source of the flooding technique may have been the method of Stampfl and Levis (1968) which the authors termed implosion therapy; by this technique the patient with a phobic neurosis is encouraged to re-experience as vividly as possible, and with all the attendant emotion, the circumstances surrounding the original conditioning event. To this extent the technique is similar to the abreactive treatment used for battle neuroses whereby the soldier was encouraged to re-experience the fear associated with the trauma. However, implosion therapy places emphasis on less obvious aversive situations such as castration danger and oedipal conflicts when these are thought to have caused the emotional state in which the neurotic symptoms had their origin; whilst imagining a scene associated with the situation the patient is strongly encouraged to experience emotions such as disgust or guilt as well as anxiety. Stampfl and Levis include their technique among the behavioural therapies since it is based upon and committed to a learning model of psychopathology although it is not purely symptom directed and does not deny the relevance of traditional psychodynamic approaches.

Marks (1972) has pointed out that flooding is not a single behavioural technique but is composed of a wide range of overlapping procedures:

> Common to all the methods is the principle of confronting the patient with the stimuli which distress him until he gets used to them and/or the evoking of intense emotion during treatment. The confrontation can take place in various ways. It can occur in a patient's imagination or in real life, individually or in groups, aided by instructions that are tape-recorded or delivered by a live therapist. It may last for a few seconds or many hours, be intermittent or continuous; escape may be allowed or curtailed, anxiety minimized or deliberately provoked, the distressing situation and unrelated events less or more elaborated upon, and therapeutic expectancies and instructions varied. The term flooding is best restricted to those forms of confrontation that evoke intense emotion. When exposure to a phobic situation is very slow and graduated, with but minimum tension, desensitisation is the most relevant term.

Reports on flooding techniques appeared with increasing frequency in the early 1970s (*inter alia*: Marks, Boulougouris, and Marset, 1971; Watson, Gaind, and Marks, 1971). In general the reports were enthusiastic about the techniques which were found to be effective, not only in the treatment of specific phobias but also in the agoraphobic syndrome which had previously responded less well to systematic desensitization. The study by Marks and his colleagues found flooding to be superior to desensitization in patients with high levels of anxiety but Gelder *et al.* (1973) were unable to confirm this conclusion. Hand, Lamontagne, and Marks (1974) found that the treatment of agoraphobia by direct exposure to anxiety in groups was followed by better long-term results if the patients had been involved in symptom-centred group discussions; Teasdale *et al.* (1977) failed to confirm the large overall and continuing improvement reported by Hand and his colleagues but concluded that treatment in cohesive groups was, none the less, one of the most cost-effective psychological treatments for agoraphobia. However, so far as this latter factor is concerned the greatest cost effectiveness must surely be that of Weeks (1973) for in her method of 'remote direction' patients are not seen by the therapist but carry out a programme of self-treatment with the aid of pamphlets and tape-recordings.

In view of the heterogeneity of patients suffering from phobic neurosis together with the imponderable variable of therapist effectiveness it is not possible at the present time to state with certainty what might be the most effective technique for any particular anxiety-based disorder. A useful review of the present position regarding behavioural and other treatments for agoraphobia has been made by Rohs and Noyes (1978). It is therefore necessary that the behavioural psychotherapist should be acquainted with a variety of techniques and to be prepared to select the one which appears to be most acceptable on many grounds, the chief of which is his personal competence with the technique. In a comparison of three behavioural techniques for the treatment of social phobia, Shaw (1979) concluded that cost effectiveness and patient acceptability were also of importance and that, for her patients, flooding was low on acceptability and social skills training was costly—therefore, given similar outcome of the methods, systematic desensitization was the treatment of choice.

Pharmacotherapy

The use of drugs in the setting of a therapeutic programme for the management of anxiety-based neuroses can often be dramatically successful but is widely misapplied. The prevalent practice of continuous prescription of the benzodiazepine sedative drugs has nothing to recommend it; at best such prescriptions may make the patient more comfortable for a short period of time but it is probable that habituation to the effect of the drug soon takes place and the continued prescription has only the disadvantages of an enormous cost to the tax payer and the risk of inducing a true drug dependence state. The latter risk is usually discounted until actual evidence for it begins to accumulate as it did with the barbiturate drugs. The barbiturates were replaced, as the popular sedative of the time, by meprobamate which, through skilful promotion, gained rapid ascendancy in the early 1950s. This drug was assumed to be an effective 'treatment' for anxiety and to be non-toxic but after some years it was found that, as with the barbiturates, habituation, addiction, and even withdrawal fits could occur. An account of the rise and fall of the drug has been given by Greenblatt and Shader (1971). They concluded:

> The history of the tranquillizer meprobamate illustrates how factors other than scientific evidence may determine physicians' patterns of drug use. Forceful advertising and publicity, an attitude of general optimism and uncontrolled studies with favourable results combined to elevate meprobamate to the position of America's magical cure-all tranquilliser. This drug remains in wide use despite a large body of sound scientific evidence which questions its efficacy. Today, easy pharmacological solutions to the stresses and tensions of life are often sought in place of more effective forms of mastery.

Meprobamate has now lost pride of place as the fashionable sedative to the benzodiazepines. These drugs produce such vast financial returns to the pharmaceutical industry that 'new' varieties of the same basic molecule appear in rapid succession (Tyrer, 1974) and yet it has not been shown, in any convincing manner, that the newer benzodiazepine drugs are any more effective than their forerunners (Lader, Bond, and James, 1974). Furthermore, the familiar evidence is beginning to emerge that true withdrawal syndromes may occur even with therapeutic doses of benzodiazepine drugs (Leading Article, *The Lancet*, 1979).

In acute severe generalized anxiety sedative drugs may be justified for a strictly limited period of time; they may also be effective in helping a patient to overcome a phobic state so long as he clearly understands that the drug is prescribed in order to help him to face up to his anxiety and should *only* be taken when he has every intention of attempting to enter the feared situation. Unfortunately, the conventional manner of prescribing the drugs on a regular basis may have the reverse of a therapeutic effect. Abrahamson (1976) in a study of the fallacies of drug prescribing remarks:

> Sedative drugs . . . interfere with problem and conflict resolution and are likely to discourage patients from attempting these tasks and their doctors from bothering to support them in doing so. The use of medication as a simplistic alternative, rather than as an adjunct to other forms of treatment is therefore made more likely.

Michael Balint (1964) in *The doctor, his patient and the illness* has analysed the process whereby a pill becomes the token of the doctor's interest; in the majority of cases this is how sedative drugs are in fact used, but they are tokens not without their dangers. Among the dangers are the possibility of inducing a state of irritability, referred to in the next chapter, and finally there is the real danger of the potentiation of the effect of alcohol; a standard work on the side-effect of drugs (Meyler and Herxheimer, 1972) states that with diazepam there is a summation effect of diazepam with alcohol and that patients prescribed such drugs should be warned to take alcohol in moderation and to take none before driving. It seems that this essential information is not always issued with prescriptions of sedative drugs and tragedy may occur by default. More recently this warning has been repeated by the Committee on the Review of Medicines (1980).

Sedative drugs, such as the benzodiazepines, will be ineffective if there is an affective disorder underlying the marked anxiety-based symptoms. The presence of such a disorder requires the prescription of an antidepressant drug, and the underlying rationale for the use of antidepressants in anxiety-based neuroses has been given earlier in the present chapter. Kelly *et al.* (1970) reported their experience of the use of antidepressant drugs in the treatment of nearly 200 adults and 50 children suffering from phobic neurosis; although the report was not based upon a double-blind trial and was, at the time, subjected to strong criticism, nevertheless the accumulated experience of these clinicians testified to the probability that both tricyclic anti-depressants and drugs of the monoamine oxidase inhibitor group had some specific effects, at least in some varieties of phobic neurosis. A later trial (Tyrer, Candy, and Kelly, 1973a) confirmed that phenelzine, a drug of the MAO inhibitor group, was effective in some phobic neuroses, particularly in agoraphobia and social phobias, whilst in the USA the earlier observation of Klein (1964) of the therapeutic role of imipramine in one type of anxiety neurosis was confirmed in a trial of the treatment of phobic neurosis (Zitrin, Klein, and Woerner, 1978). This group of workers pointed out that many patients suffering from anxiety-based neuroses experience marked side-effects after taking antidepressants; tolerance and compliance is increased by prescribing the drugs in a low dosage initially and gradually increasing the dose towards the therapeutic range over a period of a few weeks. In a further report, Zitrin *et al.* (1976) considered that the presence of severe panic attacks, particularly in the agoraphobic syndrome, was indicative of an underlying affective disorder and until this was brought under control with appropriate drug therapy, behaviour therapy would be ineffective. This observation appears to be soundly based and if there is a strong suspicion of the presence of an affective disorder there can be no justification for proceeding to a time-consuming psychotherapeutic procedure, which will probably prove ineffective, until a thorough attempt has been made to relieve the core symptoms with antidepressant drugs.

A further important group of drugs which have been established as having a role in the management of some anxiety-based neuroses are the beta-adrenergic blocking drugs. Since the first report of the use of propranolol in the treatment of anxiety states (Granville-Grossman and Turner, 1966) there has been some further research which is summarized by Tyrer (1979) who concludes that the patients who are most likely to derive benefit from such drugs are those with marked somatic symptoms of anxiety, a conclusion which is predictable from the physiological effects of beta-blockade; such patients are more likely to be encountered in general practice and in general medical clinics than in psychiatric clinics.

It may be stressed once again that if drugs are to be used in the treatment of anxiety it should only be as part of an overall therapeutic approach to the patient and his problems.

Psychosurgery

Finally, there are a small number of patients who have suffered from chronic anxiety states for many years and who have remained unresponsive to the whole gamut of therapeutic procedures; their state seems to be unrelated to any situational stress although their disorder will have brought much stress in its train. Their lives may be an agonizing experience both for themselves and for their relatives; in Burton's words: 'No rack, no torture like unto it.' For such patients psychosurgery may produce lasting relief, and, with modern surgical techniques, few if any undesirable effects. Such patients should not be denied the chance of an assessment by a psychiatrist and neurosurgeon who are experienced in the field. Earp (1979) recommends that consideration for psychosurgery should not be withheld until an extreme state of chronicity has been reached but should be offered to patients who, on the basis of an ill-sustained response to a previous course of treatment and the presence of good premorbid personality show positive indications that they might benefit from psychosurgery.

At present there is no definite indication as to which of the variety of modern techniques will produce the best results in anxiety states. Göktepe, Young, and Bridges (1975), using the technique of stereotactic subcaudate tractotomy found, in a follow-up study of over $2\frac{1}{2}$ years that, of 17 patients suffering from chronic anxiety states, 9 had recovered, 4 were improved, and in 4 patients the condition was unchanged. Using the stereotactic limbic leucotomy Mitchell-Heggs, Kelly, and Richardson (1976) found, in a 16-month follow-up of 15 patients suffering from chronic anxiety states, that 4 had recovered, 6 were improved, in 3 the condition was unchanged, and in 2 patients the patients' condition was reported as being worse. It would therefore appear that for chronic anxiety states the results of the first series from The Brook General Hospital, London may be better than those of the second series from Atkinson Morley's Hospital, London but there can be no certainty in the matter; however, both studies point to a worthwhile rate of improvement in patients with otherwise intractable illness.

A NOTE ON DEPERSONALIZATION

Depersonalization is a not uncommon experience which occurs in the healthy as well as in morbid states both of organic brain disease and a variety of functional psychiatric disorders. A Leading Article in the *British Medical Journal* (1972) defined it as follows:

> Depersonalization is a strange, complex and essentially private experience, one characteristic of which is the individual's difficulty in communicating a comprehensible account of it. A prominent feature of the experience is a feeling of change involving either or both the inner and the outer worlds and carrying with it a vague but uncomfortable sense of unfamiliarity. The description 'unreal' or 'detached' is usually accepted, but the experience varies greatly between individuals and between attacks. . . . The patient always uses an 'as if' qualification in his often bizarre descriptions of the experience, and one of the serious risks of the condition is that it may be misunderstood and a more malign significance be attributed to it.

The most thorough review of depersonalization was carried out by Sedman (1970) who quoted Mayer-Gross that depersonalization is a pre-formed functional response of the brain. The area of the brain involved is probably the limbic system which is concerned with integration of experience, memory, and mood; of all the organic syndromes, it is most frequently encountered in the aura preceding the fit of temporal lobe epilepsy. The investigations which have been carried out of records of the experience in healthy populations were summarized by Sedman, who concluded that a high proportion of young adults experience depersonalization at some time and the experience is frequently associated with conditions likely to produce slight alteration in consciousness, anxiety-producing situations, affective change, and sadness. The experience may also be induced by the drug LSD and artificially induced states of sensory deprivation and fatigue. Since the time of Sedman's review, Myers and Grant (1972) conducted another investigation in a student population and found that the experience was significantly associated with mild agoraphobia and recent disturbances in emotional health in females.

In phobic patients referred to a psychiatric clinic depersonalization is frequently described as occurring at the height of a panic attack and this fact, together with records of the experience in the dying and in battle fatigue, leads to the speculation that the pre-formed mechanism is, on occasions, a psychic defence mechanism which enables the individual to cope with extreme anxiety. Roth (1959) recorded depersonalization as a frequent symptom associated with phobic anxiety states following calamitous circumstances and both persistent (Shorvon, 1946) and episodic (Davison, 1964) depersonalization has been recorded in clinic populations with little other evidence of major psychiatric disorder. The experience may also precede a schizophrenic illness and recently Koehler (1979) has drawn attention to the experience of 'influenced' depersonalization as part of the passivity continuum of that disorder.

Depersonalization is therefore an experience which occurs in health and in disease, in organic neurological disorders and functional psychiatric syndromes, and in 'neurotic' as well as 'psychotic' disorders. A note of caution about eliciting the symptom has been sounded by Edwards and Angus (1972); a high proportion of individuals will reply in the affirmative to the question: 'Have you ever felt unreal?' but this reply may not indicate that they have experienced depersonalization. The clinician may be most certain of the presence of the symptom when the patient gives an unsolicited account of the strange and uncomfortable experience of unreality.

References

*ABRAHAMSON, D. (1976). Psychotropic drug use: fallacies and a paradox. *Psychol. Med.* **6**, 529–31.

AGRAS, W. S., CHAPIN, H. N., and OLIVEAU, D. (1972). The natural history of phobia. *Archs gen. Psychiat.* **26**, 315–17.

—— SYLVESTER, D., and OLIVEAU, D. (1969). The epidemiology of common fears and phobias. *Comp. Psychiat.* **10**, 151–6.

ANDREWS, J. D. (1966). Psychotherapy of phobias. *Psychol. Bull.* **66**, 455–80.

BALINT, M. (1964). *The doctor, his patient and the illness.* Pitman Medical, Tunbridge Wells.

BERG, I., BUTLER, A., and HALL, G. (1976). The outcome of school phobia. *Br. J. Psychiat.* **128**, 80–5.

—— and PRITCHARD, J. (1974). Psychiatric illness in the mothers of school phobic adolescents. *Br. J. Psychiat.* **125**, 466–7.

*BLACKWELL, B. (1976). Treatment adherence. *Br. J. Psychiat.* **129**, 513–31.

*British Medical Journal (1972). Depersonalization syndromes. Leading article. *Br. med. J.* **iv**, 378.

BUGLASS, D., CLARKE, J., HENDERSON, A. S., KREITMAN, N., and PRESLEY, A. S. (1977). A study of agoraphobic housewives. *Psychol. Med.* **7**, 73–86.

BURTON, Robert. *The anatomy of melancholy.* (Based on the posthumously published 6th edn.) Translated and edited by Floyd Dell and Paul Jordan-Smith. Tudor Publishing Company, New York (1927).

CAUTELA, J. H. (1965). Desensitization and insight. *Behav. Res. Ther.* **3**, 59–64.

*CHESSER, E. S. (1976). Behaviour therapy: recent trends and current practice. *Br. J. Psychiat.* **129**, 289–307.

CLANCY, J., NOYES, R., HOENK, P. R., and SLYMEN, D. J. (1978). Secondary depression in anxiety neurosis. *J. nerv. ment. Dis.* **166**, 846–50.

*COMMITTEE ON THE REVIEW OF MEDICINES (1980). Systematic review of benzodiazepines. *Br. med. J.* **i**, 910–12.

DAVISON, K. (1964). Episodic depersonalization. *Br. J. Psychiat.* **110**, 505–13.

DOLLARD, J. and MILLER, N. E. (1950). *Personality and psychotherapy.* McGraw Hill, New York.

DOWNING, R. W. and RICKELS, K. (1974). Mixed anxiety-depression. *Archs gen. Psychiat.* **30**, 312–20.

EARP, J. D. (1979). Psychosurgery, the position of the Canadian Psychiatric Association. *Can. J. Psychiat.* **24**, 353–65.

EDWARDS, J. G. and ANGUS, J. W. S. (1972). Depersonalization. *Br. J. Psychiat.* **120**, 242–4.

ERRERA, P. (1962). Some historical aspects of the concept phobia. *Psychiatr. Q.* **36**, 325–36.

EYSENCK, H. J. and RACHMAN, S. (1965). *The causes and cures of neurosis.* Routledge and Kegan Paul, London.

FRANKL, V. E. (1960). Paradoxical intention. *Am. J. Psychother.* **14**, 520–35.

FRANK, J. D. (1961). *Persuasion and healing.* Oxford University Press, London; Johns Hopkins Press, Baltimore.

FREUD, S. (1895). Obsessions and phobias. In *The standard edition of the complete psychological works*, Vol. 3 (ed. J. Strachey). Hogarth Press, London.

—— (1909). Analysis of a phobia in a five-year old boy. In *The standard edition of the complete psychological works*, Vol. 10 (ed. J. Strachey). Hogarth Press, London.

—— (1917). Lines of advance in psychoanalytic theory. In *The standard edition of the complete psychological works*, Vol. 17 (ed. J. Strachey). Hogarth Press, London.

—— (1933). Anxiety and instinctual life. In *The standard edition of the complete psychological works*, Vol. 22 (ed. J. Strachey). Hogarth Press, London.

FROMMER, E. A. (1968). Depression in childhood. In *Recent developments in affective disorders* (ed. A. Coppen and A. Walk) *British Journal of Psychiatry* Special Publication, No. 2. Headley Bros, Ashford.

GARMANY, G. (1956). Anxiety states. *Br. med. J.* **i**, 943–6.

GELDER, M. G. (1979). Behaviour therapy as self-control. In *Current themes in psychiatry* (ed. R. N. Gaind and B. L. Hudson). Macmillan, London.

—— BANCROFT, J. H. J., GATH, D. H., JOHNSTON, D. W., MATHEWS, A. M., and SHAW, P. M. (1973). Specific and non-specific factors in behaviour therapy. *Br. J. Psychiat.* **123**, 445–62.

GÖKTEPE, E. O., YOUNG, L. B., and BRIDGES, P. K. (1975). Stereotactic subcaudate tractotomy: a further review. *Br. J. Psychiat.* **126**, 270–80.

GRANVILLE-GROSSMAN, K. L. and TURNER, P. (1966). The effect of propranolol on anxiety. *Lancet* i, 788–90.

GREENBLATT, D. J. and SHADER, R. I. (1971). Meprobamate: a study of irrational drug use. *Am. J. Psychiat.* **127**, 33–9.

GURNEY, C., ROTH, M., GARSIDE, R. F., KERR, T. A., and SCHAPIRA, K. (1972). The relationship between anxiety states and depressive illness – 2. *Br. J. Psychiat.* **121**, 162–6.

HAFNER, R. J. (1977). The husbands of agoraphobic women and their influence on outcome. *Br. J. Psychiat.* **131**, 289–94.

HAND, I., LAMONTAGNE, Y., and MARKS, I. M. (1974). Group exposure (flooding) *in vivo* for agoraphobics. *Br. J. Psychiat.* **124**, 588–602.

HAYS, P. (1964). Modes of onset of psychotic depression. *Br. med. J.* ii, 779–84.

*HERSOV, L. (1977). School refusal. In *Child psychiatry, modern approaches* (ed. M. Rutter and L. Hersov). Blackwell Scientific Publications, Oxford.

JARRETT, E. J. and SCHNURR, R. (1979). Phobias and depression: clinical and psychometric aspects. *J. Behav. Ther. Exp. Psychiat.* **10**, 167–71.

JONES, E. (1964). *The life and work of Sigmund Freud.* Pelican Books, Harmondsworth.

JONES, M. C. (1924). The elimination of children's fears. *J. exp. Psychol.* **7**, 382–90.

KELLY, D., GUIRGUIS, W., FROMMER, E., MITCHELL-HEGGS, N., and SARGANT, W. (1970). The treatment of phobic states with antidepressants. *Br. J. Psychiat.* **116**, 387–98.

KERR, T. A., ROTH, M., SCHAPIRA, K., and GURNEY, C. (1972). The assessment and prediction of outcome in affective disorders. *Br. J. Psychiat.* **121**, 167–74.

KING, A. (1962). Phenelzine treatment of Roth's calamity syndrome. *Med. J. Aust.* i, 879–83.

KLEIN, D. F. (1964). Differentiation of two drug-responsive anxiety syndromes. *Psychopharmacologia* **5**, 397–408.

*KOEHLER, K. (1979). First rank symptoms of schizophrenia: questions concerning clinical boundaries. *Br. J. Psychiat.* **134**, 236–48.

KRÄUPL TAYLOR, F. (1966). *Psychopathology, its causes and symptoms.* Butterworth, London.

LADER, M. H. and MARKS, I. M. (1971). *Clinical anxiety.* Heinemann, London.

—— BOND, A. J., and JAMES, D. C. (1974). Clinical comparison of anxiolytic drug therapy. *Psychol. Med.* **4**, 381–7.

The Lancet (1976). Psychotherapy vs. behaviour therapy. Leading article. *Lancet* i, 1225–6.

*—— (1979). Benzodiazepine withdrawal. Leading article. *Lancet* i, 196.

LEWIS, A. J. (1966). Psychological medicine. In *Price's Textbook of the practice of medicine*, 10th edn (ed. Sir Ronald Bodley Scott). Oxford University Press, London.

—— (1970). The ambiguous word 'anxiety'. *Int. J. Psychiat.* **9**, 62–79.

LIEF, H. I. (1955). Sensory associations in the selection of phobic objects. *Psychiatry* **18**, 331–8.

MALLESON, N. (1959). Panic and phobia. *Lancet* **i**, 225–7.

MAPOTHER, E. (1926). Discussion on manic-depressive psychosis. *Br. med. J.* **ii**, 877–9.

MARKS, I. M. (1969). *Fears and phobias.* Heinemann, London.

—— (1972). Perspective on flooding. *Semin. Psychiat.* **4**, 129–38.

—— and GELDER, M. G. (1965). A controlled retrospective study of behaviour therapy in phobic patients. *Br. J. Psychiat.* **111**, 561–73.

—— (1966). Different ages of onset in varieties of phobia. *Am. J. Psychiat.* **123**, 218–21.

*—— BOULOUGOURIS, J. C., and MARSET, P. (1971). Flooding versus desensitization in the treatment of phobic patients. *Br. J. Psychiat.* **119**, 353–75.

MENDEL, J. G. C. and KLEIN, D. F. (1969). Anxiety attacks with subsequent agoraphobia. *Comp. Psychiat.* **10**, 190–5.

MENDELS, J., WEINSTEIN, N., and COCHRANE, C. (1972). The relationship between anxiety and depression. *Archs gen. Psychiat.* **27**, 649–53.

MEYER, V. and GELDER, M. G. (1963). Behaviour therapy and phobic disorders. *Br. J. Psychiat.* **109**, 19–28.

MEYLER, L. and HERXHEIMER, A. (1972). *The side-effects of drugs.* Excerpta Medica, Amsterdam.

MILLER, N. E. (1948). Studies of fear as an acquirable drive. *J. exp. Psychol.* **38**, 89–95.

MITCHELL-HEGGS, N., KELLY, D., and RICHARDSON, A. (1976). Stereotactic limbic leucotomy—a follow-up. *Br. J. Psychiat.* **128**, 226–40.

MULLANEY, J. A. and TRIPPETT, C. J. (1979). Alcohol dependence and phobias. *Br. J. Psychiat.* **135**, 565–74.

MYERS, D. H. and GRANT, G. (1972). A study of depersonalization in students. *Br. J. Psychiat.* **121**, 59–65.

OLLEY, M. and McALLISTER, H. (1974). A comment on the treatment analogues for phobic anxiety states. *Psychol. Med.* **4**, 463–70.

*POLLITT, J. and YOUNG, J. (1971). Anxiety state or masked depression? A study based on the action of monoamine oxidase inhibitors. *Br. J. Psychiat.* **119**, 143–9.

PRUSOFF, B. and KLERMAN, G. L. (1974). Differentiating depressed from anxious neurotic patients. *Archs gen. Psychiat.* **30**, 302–9.

ROBERTS, A. H. (1964). 'The housebound housewife'. *Br. J. Psychiat.* **110**, 191–7.

*ROHS, R. G. and NOYES, R. (1978). Agoraphobia: newer treatment approaches. *J. nerv. ment. Dis.* **166**, 701–8.

*ROTH, M. (1959). The phobic anxiety depersonalization syndrome. *Proc. R. Soc. Med.* **52**, 587–96.

—— GURNEY, C., GARSIDE. R. F., and KERR, T. A. (1972). Studies in the classification of affective disorder. *Br. J. Psychiat.* **121**, 147–61.

SCHAPIRA, K., KERR. T. A., and ROTH, M. (1970). Phobias and affective illness. *Br. J. Psychiat.* **117**, 25–32.

—— ROTH, M., KERR, T. A., and GURNEY, C. (1972). The prognosis of affective disorders: the differentiation of anxiety states from depressive illness. *Br. J. Psychiat.* **121**, 175–81.

*SEDMAN, G. (1970). Theories of depersonalization: a reappraisal. *Br. J. Psychiat.* **117**, 1–14.

SHAFER, S. (1975). Agoraphobia. *Br. med. J.* **i**, 40.

*SHAW, P. (1979). A comparison of three behaviour therapies in the treatment of social phobia. *Br. J. Psychiat.* **134**, 620–3.

SHORVON, H. J. (1946). The depersonalization syndrome. *Proc. R. Soc. Med.* **39**, 779–85.

SLOANE, H. B., STAPLES, F. R., CRISTOL, A. H., YORKSTON, N. J., and WHIPPLE, K. (1975). *Psychotherapy versus behavior therapy.* Harvard University Press, Cambridge, Massachusetts.

SNAITH, R. P. (1968). A clinical investigation of phobias. *Br. J. Psychiat.* **114**, 673–97.

—— BRIDGES, G. W. K., and HAMILTON, M. (1976). The Leeds scales for the self-assessment of anxiety and depression. *Br. J. Psychiat.* **128**, 156–65.

—— CONSTANTOPOULOS, A. A., JARDINE, M. Y., and McGUFFIN, P. (1978). A clinical scale for the self-assessment of irritability. *Br. J. Psychiat.* **132**, 164–71.

SOLYOM, L., BECK, P., SOLYOM, C., and HUGEL, R. (1974). Some etiological factors in phobic neurosis. *Can. Psychiat. Ass. L.* **19**, 69–78.

STAMPFL, T. G. and LEVIS, D. J. (1968). Implosive therapy—a behavioural therapy? *Behav. Res. Ther.* **6**, 31–6.

TEASDALE, J. D., WALSH, P. A., LANCASHIRE, M., and MATHEWS, A. M. (1977). Group exposure for agoraphobics: a replication study. *Br. J. Psychiat.* **130**, 186–93.

TERHUNE, W. B. (1949). The phobic syndrome. *Archs Neurol. Psychiat.* **62**, 162–72.

TRUAX, C. B. and MITCHELL, K. M. (1971). Research on certain therapist interpersonal skills in relation to outcome. In *Handbook of psychotherapy and behaviour change* (ed. A. E. Bergin and S. L. Garfield). Wiley, New York.

TYRER, P. (1974). The benzodiazepine bonanza. *Lancet* **ii**, 709–10.

—— (1979). Anxiety states. In *Recent advances in clinical psychiatry*, Vol. 3 (ed. K. Granville-Grossman). Churchill Livingstone, Edinburgh.

—— and TYRER, S. (1974). School refusal, truancy and adult neurotic illness. *Psychol. Med.* **4**, 416–21.

—— CANDY, J., and KELLY, D. (1973a). Phenelzine in phobic anxiety: a controlled trial. *Psychol. Med.* **3**, 120–4.

————— (1973b). A study of the clinical effects of phenelzine and placebo in the treatment of phobic anxiety. *Psychopharmacologia* **32**, 237–54.

WALKER, L. (1959). The prognosis for affective illness with overt anxiety. *J. Neurol. Neurosurg. Psychiat.* **22**, 338–41.

WATSON, J. B. (1930). *Behaviourism.* Kegan Paul, Trench and Trubner, London.

*WATSON, J. P., GAIND, R., and MARKS, I. M. (1971). Prolonged exposure—a rapid treatment for phobias. *Br. med. J.* **i**, 13–15.

WEEKES, C. (1973). A practical treatment for agoraphobia. *Br. med. J.* **ii**, 469–71.

WOLPE, J. (1958). *Psychotherapy by reciprocal inhibition.* Stanford University Press, California.

—— (1964). Behaviour therapy in complex neurotic states. *Br. J. Psychiat.* **110**, 28–34.

WORLD HEALTH ORGANIZATION (1978). *Mental disorders: glossary and guide to their classification in accordance with the ninth revision of the International Classification of Diseases.* Geneva.

YOUNG, J. P. R., FENTON, G. W., and LADER, M. H. (1971). The inheritance of neurotic traits; a twin study of The Middlesex Hospital questionnaire. *Br. J. Psychiat.* **119**, 393–8.

ZITRIN, C. M., KLEIN, D. F., and WOERNER, M. G. (1978). Behaviour therapy, supportive therapy, imipramine and phobias. *Archs gen. Psychiat.* **35**, 307–6.

———— LINDEMANN, C., TOBAK, P., ROCK. M., KAPLAN, J. H., and GANZ, V. H. (1976). Comparison of short term treatment regimes in phobic patients. In *Evaluation of psychological therapies: psychotherapies, behaviour therapies, drug therapies and their interaction* (ed. R. L. Spitzer and D. F. Klein). Johns Hopkins University Press, Baltimore, Maryland.

2

Depressive neurosis

THE glossary to the 9th revision of the *International classification of diseases* (WHO, 1978) defines neurotic depression as follows:

> 300.4   A neurotic disorder characterized by disproportionate depression which has *usually* recognizably ensued on a distressing experience; it does not include among its features delusions or hallucinations, and there is *often* a preoccupation with the psychic trauma which preceded the illness, e.g. loss of a cherished person or possession. Anxiety is also *frequently* present and mixed states of anxiety and depression should be included here. The distinction between depressive neurosis and psychosis should be made not only upon the degree of depression but also on the presence or absence of other neurotic and psychotic characteristics and upon the degree of disturbance of the patient's behaviour. — (Italics added)

This definition is couched in such general terms that the user is left free to employ the category as widely, or as narrowly, as he chooses. The only definite statement in the whole definition is, that if delusions or hallucinations are present, then the disorder may not be classified as neurotic depression.

It is not certain when the word depression was first used in a psychopathological context, but in 1883, in the first edition of his *Lehrbuch*, Kraepelin referred to *Depressionzustände* (depressive states) and in 1896, in a later edition of the same work, the term *manisch-depressive Irresein* (manic-depressive psychosis) was introduced. Before 1909 the word appeared only once in the index of the *Journal of Mental Science* (the forerunner of the *British Journal of Psychiatry*); this was in a review of Clouston's Annual Report on Morningside Hospital, where it was noted that: 'States of depression are becoming as frequent as states of exaltation as causes for admission to the asylum' (Alexander Walk; personal communication). Until the present century, severe depressive states were usually called melancholia but the American psychiatrist, Adolf Meyer, was dissatisfied with this term and its implication that the condition was a physical disease arising from some disorder of the bile. In 1905, as a discussant at a symposium on classification, he made a plea that the term melancholia should be abandoned and replaced by depression:

> If, instead of melancholia, we applied the term depression to the whole class, it would designate in an unassuming way exactly what was meant by the common use of the word melancholia and nobody would doubt that for medical purposes the term would have to be amplified so as to denote the kind of depression. In the large group of depressions we would naturally distinguish our cases according to etiology, the symptom-complex, the course of the disease and the results.

The adoption of the term, which Meyer advocated, was soon widespread but did not bring in its wake the hoped-for clarification of the issues. In fact the reverse was the case for much of the present confusion has arisen out of the use of a word which has no precise meaning and which moreover, is employed in many different contexts and senses. In everyday usage depression is taken to mean a variety of unpleasant moods including a feeling of sadness, a feeling of dejection, an experience of hopelessness or pessimism and a lowering of the responses of pleasure and mirth, all of which, whether they occur separately or together, have a recognizable origin in some adversity and are therefore considered to be justified and normal moods. In the context of psychopathology the word depression is used for a similar variety of moods which are considered to be symptoms of many psychiatric disorders but the moods are now usually more intense and prolonged and may not be explained in terms of adversity. Furthermore, depression is employed as a nosological category although usually preceded by some such term as 'neurotic', 'reactive', 'exogenous', 'psychotic', 'primary', or 'secondary'. The present situation is rather as if the one word 'panting' was used for normal shortness of breath after running up a flight of steps, for dyspnoea experienced when attempting to lie flat in bed, and for the disorders of asthma and congestive cardiac failure.

The American psychiatrist Beck (1967), posed the following questions:

1. Is depression merely an exaggeration of the normal mood state or is it qualitatively different?
2. Is depression a well-defined clinical entity or merely a collection of diverse disorders?

3. Is depression a reaction, in the Meyerian sense, or a disease in the Kraepelinian sense?

4. Is depression primarily the result of psychological conflict or is it primarily a manifestation of biological disorder?

He pointed out that there are no universally accepted answers to these questions and nor, it appears, can there ever be unless terminology in this area becomes more precisely defined. However, since this is unlikely to come about in the near future we must attempt to be aware of the variety of concepts and hope that clinicians and investigators may become rather more precise in their communications between themselves and the public than at the present time.

In order to be clearer about the difficulties surrounding the concept of depressive neurosis a brief survey of the attempts at definition and differentiation from other depressive disorders will now be undertaken.

THE DIFFERENTIATION OF DEPRESSIVE NEUROSIS FROM OTHER DEPRESSIVE DISORDERS

At the time when the term melancholia was beginning to fall out of diagnostic fashion psychiatrists were emerging from their closed institutions and were seeing patients with less severe forms of mental disorder than would require compulsory admission to mental hospitals. It then became necessary to distinguish severe depressive states from less severe forms; the term psychosis was generally appended to the former and neurosis to the latter. Depressive neurosis and depressive psychosis were sometimes considered to be distinct disorders with different causes and prognoses but Mapother (1926) at The Maudsley Hospital did not accept this view:

> The distinction between what are termed neuroses and psychoses has really grown out of practical differences, particularly as regards certification and asylum treatment. It has been customary to call those types and degrees of mental disorder which rarely call for such measures by the name of neuroses. I can find no basis for this distinction; neither insight, nor co-operation in treatment nor susceptibility to psychotherapy will serve. . . . The view that neurosis and depressive psychosis represent a continuum and that both are associated with lasting bodily anomalies is not, of course, in the least inconsistent with believing that the traces of unpleasant experience are one of the principle causes of both. . . . It would need an extreme degree of clinical blindness to ignore the fact that,

in a very large proportion of both neuroses and psychoses of the depressive type, the attack is directly related to stress, and as a rule the exact emotional anomaly corresponds to a morbid protraction of what circumstances would naturally cause.

Thus colours were nailed to the mast of the unitary, or continuum, view of the nature of depressive disorder and a few psychiatrists sailing under the separatist flag replied briefly, but angrily, in subsequent issues of the *British Medical Journal*.

A few years later, at Guy's Hospital, Gillespie (1929) had introduced the term 'reactive' depression; by the use of this adjective he did not imply that the disorder was a reaction to circumstances, in the Meyerian sense, but that the mood improved, if only briefly, under certain conditions; in other words, the patient was capable of cheering up under circumstances he enjoyed such as (Gillespie instanced) a game of tennis.

Lewis, who followed Mapother at the Maudsley Hospital, was also suspicious of attempts to classify depressive disorders into discrete categories and he warned of the possible danger of classification since the treatment might become too rigid in that it was blinkered by the clinician's diagnosis. In 1938 he wrote:

> It is very probable that all the tables and classifications in terms of symptoms are nothing more than attempts to distinguish between acute and chronic, mild and severe: and where two categories alone are presented, the one — manic-depressive — gives the characteristics of acute, severe depression, the other of mild chronic depression.

However, Lewis did not entirely deny that different patterns of depressive disorder might exist but he held to the opinion that they could not be readily distinguished on symptomatological grounds, precipitation, or course of the illness. In his earlier classic and exhaustive study of 61 depressed patients treated by himself (Lewis, 1934) he concluded that, in a small group of nine patients, a particular situation appeared to be an indispensable cause for the attack although the illness could not be entirely explained by it; in another small group of ten patients he had not been able, even after extensive inquiries from many sources of information, to discover anything in the patient's environment that might be held responsible for the attack of depression. For the majority of his patients the depressive disorder was best understood in terms of an interaction between the individual and the environment, the personality structure and the stresses of life, and he pointed out that the more one knew about the patient, the more so was this view confirmed. This was a clear statement of the 'interactionalist' position, and the clinical study on which it was based must still be held in high regard for no subsequent studies have ever reported such intense detail of such a large group of patients treated by a single clinician.

The introduction of treatments, and especially electroconvulsive therapy, which were apparently effective in some depressive states but not in others, increased the need to determine which patients might be expected to respond to such treatments and which should be treated by the more time-consuming psychotherapeutic measures. Hamilton and White (1959) were the earliest investigators to apply the multivariate statistical technique of factor analysis to clinical data recorded in depressed patients; they concluded that endogenous depression differed not only quantitatively from other forms of depression but constituted a separate category, although they could not entirely justify this conclusion by acceptable levels of statistical significance. This study was followed by other inquiries and Mendels and Cochrane (1968) published a report of seven factor analytic studies carried out by five different 'schools' of psychiatrists. They pointed out that the seven studies were in agreement concerning an 'endogenous' pattern of depression characterized by psychomotor retardation, severe depression, lack of reactivity to environmental changes, loss of interest in life, visceral symptoms, insomnia in the middle part of the night, and a lack both of a tendency to self-pity and of a clear precipitant of the illness. However, Mendels and Cochrane concluded that 'endogenous' and 'reactive' patterns had not been established as distinct disorders and that the endogenous pattern might reflect a classical depressive syndrome whereas the reactive pattern might reflect a range of psychiatric disorders in which depression is one symptom accompanied by other non-depressive clinical features. The main value of their report was to point out the major failing of all investigations of this type, that of rater bias; this is the possibility, indeed the likelihood, of error introduced by an investigator who arrives at a conclusion about a patient based on one clinical feature and then unwittingly searches more diligently for other features which will support this view. Thus, if an investigator considers that there is a distinct entity of endogenous depression and if he observes psychomotor retardation in a patient he might then expend rather more effort in eliciting ideas of guilt.

In a review of the attempts to classify depression, Kendell (1976) arrived at a similar conclusion to Mendels and Cochrane and pointed out that, whilst most studies had identified a pattern which could be termed endogenous depression, few had found a contrasting pattern which could with confidence be identified as depressive neurosis or reactive depression. Kiloh *et al.* (1972) concluded that depressive neurosis is a diagnosis arrived at by exclusion of the features of endogenous depression and Foulds (1973), strongly advocating the hierarchical view of psychiatric disorder, considered that the relationship between depressive neurosis and depressive psychosis was an inclusive one, in that all patients with psychotic depressive symptoms also have neurotic depressive symptoms, but not vice versa. In a criticism of the concept of depressive neurosis, Ascher (1952) considered that the confusion about classification was a 'left-over' from the era of descriptive psychiatry and that, neither the course of the illness nor the therapeutic success of various procedures, nor the danger of suicide were consistent enough, within any one category, to justify the continued use of categorical classification. Akiskal *et al.* (1978) have listed the elements that enter into the concept of neurotic depression.

1. Contrasted to 'psychosis': preservation of reality testing, insight, and lack of psychotic symptoms such as hallucinations and delusions.

2. Mild illness: the mood disorder is considered to be less severe and in particular there is less disturbance of such physiological functions as appetite, sleep, and libido.

3. Coexistence of neurotic symptoms: although depressive symptoms dominate the clinical picture such 'neurotic' symptoms as obsessions, phobias, anxiety, and depersonalization are also present.

4. Reactivity or psychogenesis: the depression is understandable in terms of adversity.

5. Characterological depression: a life-long tendency to overreact to stress with a mood of depression.

Klerman *et al.* (1979) produced a similar list of discriminants between endogenous and neurotic depression, with the addition that unconscious conflicts were presumed to be present in the neurotic form of the disorder. They found that there was only a modest degree of overlap between these elements if depression was to be categorized by them; for instance if patients had been defined as 'endogenous' by the presence of psychotic symptoms then 37 per cent of these patients had also a clear precipitant for the illness and these defining criteria are therefore not mutually exclusive. They proposed that the term neurotic depression should be dropped and they introduced a classification based, not on discrete categories, nor a single continuum but along a series of dimensions; unfortunately for their view the majority of these six 'dimensions' cannot be considered to be true dimensions at all, but none the less the idea is a useful one and is likely in time to prove fruitful. A patient who is suffering from depression may be considered to be occupying a position in a polydimensional frame of reference. Which of the multitude of dimensions are considered will depend upon the interests of the investigator or clinician, but one of them will be the degree to which the disorder is precipitated by stress; a second will be the severity of the depression; and a third the individual's constitutional vulnerability to depression as estimated by the occurrence of the disorder in relatives. A further dimension, or set of dimensions, will be concerned with particular personality traits and other determinants of the individual's position in the polydimensional space will not be dimensions but factors such as gender and ethnic origin. The position relative to all these, and other, dimensions will determine the clinical manifestations, the actual symptoms, of the depressive disorder. One dimension which has received surprisingly little attention in studies of the phenomena of depression is that of age and yet it is probable that the age of the individual has a major influence on the type of symptoms that develop. For instance, insomnia in the last part of the night is considered to be characteristic of endogenous depression but this category is diagnosed more frequently in older people than in younger people and older people are more prone to awake early even in the absence of depression. Anxiety symptoms occur more frequently in younger people and marked anxiety as a feature of a depressive state is a feature of depression in younger people.

Paykel (1971) studied the patterns of depression by the technique of cluster analysis and identified four groups: the first was characterized by severe illness, sometimes with delusions; the second group was characterized by depression of moderate severity with marked anxiety; in the third group depression was associated with considerable hostility and the fourth group was a relatively mild illness developing on the background of personality disorder. The corresponding mean ages of these four groups were 47, 40, 34, and 29 years respectively which is at least suggestive that an age factor plays a part in the symptomatic presentation of depressive disorder. One of the few papers that have specifically dealt with the relation of age to the pattern of depression was that of Spicer, Hare, and Slater (1973); they considered that differences in symptomatology which have commonly been accepted as distinguishing neurotic from psychotic forms of depression might simply be related to age.

The probability that the manifestations of depressive disorder are partly dependent upon age raises the matter of masked and atypical forms of depression and the important question of depression in childhood. West and Dally (1959) identified a group of young adult patients with prominent neurotic symptoms, especially phobic anxiety, who responded well to treatment with the antidepressant drug iproniazid, a monoamine oxidase inhibitor; largely on the basis of this response, but also on the grounds that depressive symptomatology was present, although overshadowed by anxiety symptoms, West and Dally considered that these patients suffered from atypical depression. Another study (Pitt, 1968) led the author to conclude that a pattern of mood disorder occurring in young women following childbirth was basically depressive in nature, although the prominent symptoms were anxiety and irritability, and again the term atypical depression was proposed.

The debate as to whether depressive disorder occurs in childhood now centres around the question of how it should be recognized in prepubertal children (Welner, 1978). Graham (1974) accepted that depressive states do occur, albeit rarely. Others have emphasized the masked or atypical presentation of depression at this period of life but this concept appears to have found most favour in the United States. Lesse (1968) thought that some forms of 'acting out' and sociopathic behaviour, hypochondriacal and psychosomatic problems, and also school phobia could all be manifestations of depression in childhood. Cytryn and McKnew (1972) considered that depression in childhood frequently presented in an atypical form and its manifestations might include hyperactivity, aggressive behaviour, psychosomatic disorders, and delinquency. In Britain,

Frommer (1968) concluded, largely on the basis of response to antidepressant drugs, that some children with eneuresis and encopresis in addition to some school phobic children, were suffering from a form of depressive disorder. Kolvin and Nicol (1979) have reviewed the topic of depression in childhood.

There is therefore a range of opinion about depression in childhood which stretches from denial of its occurrence to the opposite pole in which a vast amount of emotional disorder is included in the concept. This debate would be of little more than academic interest were it not for the possibility of response of some types of disturbance to antidepressant drugs. This area of investigation deserves high priority for, if it can be established which, if any, of the disturbances of childhood respond consistently to treatment with these drugs then considerable family dysharmony, present misery and later neurotic disability could be prevented.

The recent tradition in British psychiatry has adhered to the categorical view of depressive states with little tendency of overlap between the categories and this view is supported by the influential textbook of Slater and Roth (1969). Against this view is the continuum concept, best expounded by Kendell (1969), who proposed that at either end of the continuum more or less classical examples of psychotic and neurotic depressive forms might occur and that there is no point of rarity separating the two forms but rather a continuous progression of intermediate patterns of disorder. In the rest of this chapter the topic of depressive neurosis will be considered largely from the continuum viewpoint; it would be difficult to do otherwise since many of the important and influential studies, especially in the field of psychological and social causation, have not clearly distinguished neurotic from psychotic forms of depression.

THE NATURE AND CAUSES OF DEPRESSION

As already mentioned, much of the confusion that surrounds the current concepts of depression stems from the imprecise meaning of the term. The same word 'depression' is used to cover such different mental states as transient grief, dissatisfaction with the circumstances of life, long-standing personality traits of pessimism, and agonizing dysphoric states occurring for no obvious reason. All these conditions may intermingle in a kaleidoscopic fashion so that, for instance, the frustrated and unhappy individual may develop a profound grief reaction and the constitutional pessimist may be as liable as the buoyant optimist to the development of an illness of the type that was once called melancholia.

Akiskal and McKinney (1975), in a comprehensive review of recent research into depression, pointed out that depressive disorders are conceptualized along specialized frames of reference which largely depend on the training of the investigator; those trained in academic psychology look to the prior experience of the individual as the basis for mood disorder, psychoanalysts search for intrapsychic conflicts, the medically-trained doctor may expect to find disease patterns based upon hereditarily determined biochemical disorder, and the sociologist proposes that faults in the structure of society are at the root of depressive disorder.

Loss and life change

The mental state of the grief-stricken bereaved person is similar to that of those who suffer from depression from other causes. It is therefore understandable that the concept of loss plays a central role in many theories about the nature of depression. In his essay *Mourning and melancholia* Freud (1917) developed a theory about the nature of depression but he first made a distinction between grief and depressive illness (or melancholia):

> Although grief involves grave departures from the normal attitude to life, it never occurs to us to regard it as a morbid condition and hand the mourner over to medical treatment. We rest assured that after a lapse of time it will be overcome and we look upon any interference with it as inadvisable or even harmful. . . . The distinguishing mental features of melancholia are a profoundly painful dejection, abrogation of interest in the outside world, loss of the capacity to love, inhibition of all activity, and a lowering of the self-regarding feelings to a degree that finds utterance in self-reproaches and self-revilings and culminates in a delusional expectation of punishment. This picture becomes a little more intelligible when we consider that, with one exception, the same traits are met with in grief. The fall in self-esteem is absent in grief, but otherwise the features are the same. . . . In grief the world becomes poor and empty; in melancholia it is the ego itself.

In this essay Freud developed the theory, which he attributed to Abraham, of introjected hostility as a central process in the causation of depression:

If one listens patiently to the self-accusations of the melancholiac, one cannot in the end, avoid the impression that often the most violent of them are hardly applicable to the patient himself but that, with insignificant modifications, they do fit someone else, some person whom the patient loves, has loved or ought to love. . . . So we get the key to the clinical picture by perceiving that the self-reproaches are reproaches against a loved object which have been shifted onto the patient's ego.

The view is then developed that following this process of introjection the ego is sadistically treated by the superego. The spontaneous remissions of melancholia are explained in terms of the process of reality testing, which is the same process that brings the normal grief reaction to an end.

The concept that depression is a result, either directly or after some psychic transformation, of the traumatic experience of loss is an attractive hypothesis and investigators have expended considerable effort to establish the connection. Freud insisted that the loss which resulted in melancholia might not be only that of death of a loved one but might include all those situations of being wounded, hurt, neglected, out of favour, or disappointed which would reinforce the ambivalence towards another person. However, the investigator would find it to be a formidable task to record all these states and moreover there would be no certain way of knowing which had preceded the depression and which were in fact not causative but consequent upon the altered mood. Most research has therefore concentrated upon the more obvious degrees of loss through death or separation.

Psychiatrists have frequently stressed the importance of the relationship between the child and the parent, particularly the mother, in determining the subsequent development and mental health of the individual. Melanie Klein (1948) proposed that the infant passes through a developmental stage, which she called the depressive position, which results from fear that he may destroy the mother he hates (the bad object). If he can successfully integrate this with the mother he loves (the good object) the depressive position is resolved, but in the event of failure the seeds are sown for the development of depression in later life.

Bowlby has frequently asserted that adverse effects may follow separation from, or loss of, a parent at an early age. There have been many studies of the effect of parental death on the subsequent mental health of the individual and these have been reviewed by

Granville-Grossman (1968). He drew the conclusion that there was no consistent evidence that parental deprivation was of aetiological importance in the development of depression later in life. Among the most careful of the studies which supported this conclusion was that of Munro (1966) but in the same year, Dennehy (1966) published an equally careful study which in many respects is a model for such investigations; she found an excess of male depressives who had lost their mother and of female depressives who had lost their father, and that, for both sexes, depressives had suffered a loss of either parent (in excess of the control population) between the ages of ten and fifteen years; it is of interest that these significant differences were not found if the parental loss had occurred during either of the two early five-year age periods. As Felix Brown (1966) pointed out, most children are resilient and can cope with disaster, such as the death of a parent, if the psychological and social support is good; the efficacy of the extended family, the humanity of the social services and the kindness of neighbours in helping the orphan are all of major importance for the future mental health of the child. It may be the adverse effects arising from the lack of such support rather than the actual death of the parent which leads to a proneness to depression in later life.

An alternative explanation of the link between death of a parent and later depression is generally overlooked by theorists and this is the possibility of a hereditary factor. Death during young adulthood may have occurred through suicide, in which case the proband would probably have grown up in ignorance of the true cause of his parent's death. Moreover, there is evidence that there is a shortened life-span for people suffering from neuroses in general (Sims, 1978) and from depressive illness in particular (Kerr, Schapira, and Roth, 1969).

If the early loss of a parent were not through death but due to some other cause, then the problem of ascertaining the role of the event in the development of depression is even more difficult. As Granville-Grossman pointed out, the departure of a parent from the home may have been due to affective illness in either one or other of the partners or else the patient himself might have had a distinctive premorbid personality of a type which, during his childhood, placed an undue burden on the parental relationship and contributed to the breakdown of marriage. The relationship of recent bereavement to depression has been investigated by Clayton and her colleagues

(1968; 1972). They noted that the manifestations of distress in early widowhood were not dissimilar to depressive illness: depressed mood, crying, and sleep disturbance occurred in more than half of the subjects whilst difficulty in concentration, loss of interest, anorexia, and weight loss were rather less common although they still occurred frequently. In contrast to depressive illness, the grief reaction was not more common in women than in men, it was not more often associated with a positive family history of affective disorder, and it was not more common in those who had recently been treated for depressive illness. This finding echos Freud's view, quoted earlier, that in grief the world seems a poorer place whilst in melancholia it is the ego itself which is impoverished. Clayton and her colleagues found that the only clear discriminant factor between widows who did, or did not, develop a grief reaction was the absence of a continuing close relationship with the offspring of the marriage.

Recently, life-event studies have concentrated upon a number of stressful factors, in addition to bereavement, as relevant to the genesis of depressive states. Paykel *et al.* (1969) carried out an investigation into the occurrence of significant recent events in the patient's life during the six-month period preceding the onset of the depression. They classified and grouped the events in certain ways and found that three out of the 33 events which they examined were significantly more common at the one-in-a-hundred level of significance in the depressed patients than in the control population: (a) increase in arguments with the spouse; (b) marital separation; (c) starting a new type of work. A further five events were more frequent at the one-in-twenty level of significance and these included the departure from home of a family member, change in work conditions, serious personal illness, and serious illness or death of a member of the family. Paykel and his colleagues considered the possibility that the events recorded by depressed patients may have been consequences rather than causes of the mood disturbance but did not consider that their findings had been seriously affected in this way. Nevertheless, the possibility remains; depressive disorders rarely have their onset at a definite point in time, from which a six-month period may be antedated, although there may be a time of sudden worsening of the symptoms which is incorrectly considered to be the onset of the disorder. In patients suffering from psychotic depression, Hays (1964) recorded that, prior to the onset of manifest depressive illness, there was a long period of less pronounced neurotic symptoms in a high proportion of the patients. If such symptoms were to include irritability, loss of interest, loss of libido, and an increased alcohol intake then the occurrence of events such as family arguments and the breakdown of relationships may reasonably be considered to be consequent upon the disordered mood of the proband rather than as the cause of his illness.

Hudgens, Morrison, and Barchha (1967) investigated 40 patients who had been hospitalized for affective disorder. In 60 per cent of their patients a recognizable event was associated with the depressive state but frequently depression was well established before the event occurred and events related to interpersonal discord were more likely to occur after the onset of the psychiatric disorder which suggests that they were consequent upon, rather than causative of, the depression.

Life-event research is beset by methodological traps and many of these have been enumerated by Alarcon and Covi (1972). More recently Andrews and Tennant (1978) have advised clinicians to continue to help their patients to cope with the stresses of life but to suspend judgement on what should be considered to be causal factors in depressive illness until more evidence is at hand.

Cognitive and behavioural models

The cognitive view of depression is that the disorder of mood is not the primary feature but is itself consequent on faulty thinking. Beck (1967) has developed the thesis that the mood disorder is determined by the way an individual structures his experience and that it is mediated by the way of schemas. A schema is a particular set of attitudes and beliefs through which the individual appraises and interprets his environment, other people, and himself. According to this view the individual who is prone to depression has adopted a schema, early in life, which is characterized by negative conceptions of his own worth; he acquires such a schema from personal experience, from the judgement of others, and from his identification with members of the family and with friends. Once such a schema has been formed it tends to be self-reinforcing and Beck gives the example of a child who gets the notion that he is inept as a result of being called inept by someone else; as a result he then interprets subsequent experiences in the light of this self-concept and gradually the schema becomes structuralized and remains throughout life, although it may be dormant and not manifested as depression. The onset of the depression is the result of the activation of three major cognitive patterns which are considered to be the primary triad of the disorder : a ..egative view of the world, a negative view of himself, and a negative view of the future, from which arise the symptoms of depressed mood, paralysis of the will, avoidance wishes, suicidal preoccupation, and increased dependency on others. In the light of the first component of the triad the individual interprets his interaction with his environment as representing defeat, deprivation, and disparagement. From the second component he regards himself as inadequate and unworthy so that he interprets his unpleasant experiences as being due to personal defect, and in the light of the third component of the triad he can envisage only continuing suffering and frustration. Thus, in depressive disorder the depressed mood is not the primary disturbance but is based upon a preformed schema which may not be discernible at any given period of his life but which persists in a latent state, like an explosive charge, ready to be detonated by an appropriate set of conditions.

To illustrate this, Beck cites the example of a businessman who felt inferior as a child since his classmates came from more prosperous families than himself. When, later, he was elected to a board of directors he felt that his colleagues were of a better social standing than himself and he became depressed. Events which activate the latent sense of inferiority, such as failure in work and relationships, are believed to be particularly likely to precipitate depression in the vulnerable individual and, as the depression deepens, the secondary mood change may further aggravate the faulty cognition.

Although this view of the nature of depressive illness is both coherent and plausible it remains to be proved that individuals prone to the disorder hold such negative self-concepts more frequently, or to a greater degree, than those who do not become depressed. Moreover in this theory there is the usual pitfall of confounding cause and effect. Beck considers that the depression develops in situations which lower self-esteem such as failing an examination, being jilted by a lover, being rejected by a fraternity, or being fired from a job, but it is possible that all such events are the consequence of the depressive state and not the precipitant of it.

Depressive disorders have not been subjected to the same degree of investigation from the standpoint of learning theory as have anxiety states but a prominent exception is the behavioural formulation of depression by Liberman and Raskin (1971). They put forward the view that depression results from a sudden decrease of social reinforcement for adaptive behaviour and the disorder is then maintained by contingent attention and concern from others. The authors consider that their theory also explains the paradox of depression developing in the context of success, such as promotion; old colleagues who dispensed positive feedback are no longer available and the individual must now supply reinforcement to others rather than receive it himself, a situation which is depleting. Lazarus (1968) holds similar views and states that the depressed person is virtually on an extinction trial as a result of withdrawal of significant reinforcers such as love, money, status, and prestige; depression occurring at the pinnacle of success may also be due to the loss of a significant reinforcer: the need to strive.

Seligman (1975) has recently promulgated the view that depression in man parallels the state of 'learned helplessness' produced experimentally in animals. In a series of experiments he produced this state in dogs and rats. Briefly, the dog, strapped into a harness, is exposed to the trauma of electric shocks which cannot be averted by any behaviour on the part of the animal; then, the dog is placed in a shuttle box one half of which is electrified; the naïve dog may escape the shocks by leaping over the barrier but the 'pretreated' animal simply continues to lie in the electrified zone. Outside the shuttle box the experimental dog demonstrates a submissive posture with no signs of lively excitement when approached by the experimenter. This is the state of learned helplessness. Seligman then makes the daring leap of equating depression in humans with this artificially produced state in animals. He views depressive disorder as developing on the basis of past experience of futility and inability to control those elements in his life which produce gratification and, on the basis of this, some event such as a bereavement precipitates the attack. However, as with Beck's theory, there is no demonstration that such prior experience or set of attitudes invariably precede the onset of depression in individuals vulnerable to the disorder. Seligman does not hold that his theory is valid for all the variety of disorders which are subsumed under the term depression.

McAuley (1979) has made a useful survey of behavioural views of depression and of the results of treatment based on behaviour therapy. He concluded that the reports of successfully treated cases were based upon mild disorders not representative of neurotic depressions commonly seen at psychiatric out-patient clinics and that, although the techniques have proved useful in some cases, their general clinical utility has yet to be demonstrated.

Social causes of depression

There is a growing interest in the possibility that depressive disorders are related to certain pathogenic social factors and there are good reasons to examine the relationship between a condition characterized by despondency and such factors as low social status, economic adversity, and the gulf between expectation and realization.

A major stimulus to the development of social theories has been the indisputable evidence that depression is more common in women than in men. Weissman and Klerman (1977) examined the evidence from a variety of sources and concluded that there is a female preponderance of depression of nearly two to one, at least in nations where people of European stock predominate. They consider several possible factors that may have contributed to this apparent predominance, including the greater readiness of women to seek help and the greater use of alcohol by men in the attempt to assuage depression which leads to a different labelling of the disorder. With these and other sources of error taken into account they conclude that the sex differences are real. Various explanations for the discrepancy are examined, including the possibility of an X-linked genetic factor and endocrine factors. Two psychosocial explanations were advanced: the 'social status' hypothesis and the 'learned helplessness' hypothesis. The first of these hypotheses considers that depression in women results from social discrimination which leads to legal and economic helplessness, dependency on others, low self-esteem, and low aspirations. The second hypothesis proposes that socially conditioned stereotypes produce a cognitive set against assertion which, grounded in the experience of the young girl, results in a limited response repertoire when under stress. No certain conclusions are drawn concerning these hypotheses but they do consider that one fact is established, which is that married women are more prone to depression than single, widowed, or divorced women. Marriage has a protective effect for men but the reverse is the case for women.

Pollitt (1977) also examined the possible reasons for the sex difference in the prevalence of depression. He was not impressed with social explanations and considered that the premenstrual tension and postnatal depression, possibly related to endocrine factors, contributed to the difference. He cited evidence that the most vulnerable time for the woman was from puberty to the age of 45 and that after the age of 55 the discrepancy in the prevalence of depression between the sexes disappears.

The sociologist George Brown and his colleagues have assembled evidence for the social causation of depression in women. This work has been subjected to detailed criticism by Tennant and Bebbington (1978) to which Brown (1978) replied. The interpretation of the findings of Brown and his colleagues is a very complex matter which does not necessarily lead to the conclusion that depression is a socially determined phenomenon. They have proposed that the development of a depressive disorder depends upon 'vulnerability factors', 'provoking agents', and 'symptom formation factors'. They have identified four vulnerability factors: (a) having three or more children under the age of 14 years; (b) unemployed status; (c) loss of the mother before the age of 11 years; (d) a lack of an intimate, confiding relationship with the spouse or boyfriend. However, each of these factors may be due to a number of causes. The woman who has given birth to children is subject to depression which is neither a chance event (Kendell *et al.*, 1976) nor a rare event (Pitt, 1968). The nature of postnatal depression has yet to be established and certainly a loss of social freedom, and of earning power may contribute to the mood disorder; however, an explanation of the disorder in biological terms, such as that advanced by Dalton (1971), cannot be discounted. The lack of an intimate relationship, as previously emphasized, may be the result of a depressive illness and not causative of it. Unemployed status is, of course, associated with the presence in the home of young children but may also result from the presence of a depressive disorder. Finally, the early death of the mother may, as stated earlier in the present chapter, have been caused by suicide or physical disease related to an affective disorder thus leading to alternatives to the social explanation.

The biological basis of depression

The evidence that depressive illness is fundamentally a biological disorder has been accumulating throughout the past 25 years. However, this evidence has been based upon studies of patients suffering from severe depressive states and none of it can, with certainty, be applied to the heterogeneous collection of mood disorders at present included in the single category of depressive neurosis. The evidence for the biological basis of depression is based upon the following sources:

(a) The demonstration of a genetic component in depressive psychosis;

(b) The observation that certain drugs, in particular reserpine, may precipitate a depressive illness;

(c) The growing knowledge of the neurochemical disturbances associated with depressive illness, particularly in the indoleamine and catecholamine systems of the biogenic amines;

(d) The reversal of depressive states by physical treatment, especially ECT and drugs affecting the monoamine systems quoted above;

(e) The association of depressive states with certain physical diseases such as Parkinson's disease, Cushing's syndrome, and certain viral infections.

It is not possible to review the extensive literature for any of these sources of evidence here. So far as depressive neurosis is concerned there is at present no evidence for a genetic basis (Stenstedt, 1966) but that investigation did not attempt the subdivision of depressive neurosis although the author did point out the difficulty of distinguishing between neurotic and endogenous depression. However, the observation has been made that mild or moderately severe depressive states, some accompanied by phobic anxiety symptoms (and therefore resembling the stereotype of depressive neurosis) may follow the viral disease infectious mononucleosis (Cadie, Nye, and Storey, 1976). Furthermore, there is accumulating clinical evidence that at least some patterns of neurotic depression, and especially those types accompanied by marked anxiety symptoms respond to treatment with drugs acting on the monoamine systems of the brain such as the monoamine oxidase inhibitors (Tyrer, 1976). There is, therefore, some evidence for a biological basis for some patterns of mood disorder that at present are included under the rubric of depressive neurosis.

ASPECTS OF TREATMENT

The categorical label depressive neurosis (more commonly called neurotic depression) covers a wide variety of psychopathological states, from the temporary and understandably gloomy feeling following disappointment or loss, through longstanding pessimism to mild but persistent moods of sadness and joylessness (anhedonia) accompanied by such neurotic symptoms as phobias, anxiety attacks, and irritability arising, for no obvious reason, in an individual of a previously happy temperament. The combinations are almost infinite and the arrival at the 'correct diagnosis' does not resolve the clinician's uncertainty or automatically lead to the appropriate treatment; rather, the reverse may be true and Lewis warned of the danger, in the whole area of depressive disorders, of being blinkered by the diagnosis which at first seems most appropriate to the patient's condition. There is no quick or infallible method by which the patient's experience may be understood and the only technique on which the clinician may rely is his preparedness to listen, perhaps over a period of more than one session, meanwhile curbing the impulse to prescribe either drugs or advice.

The word depression is widely used and the statement 'I feel so depressed' is not a description of a symptom but the sufferer's invitation for an exploration of his state of mind. Leff (1978) has examined the different concepts of patients and psychiatrists in the use of words such as depression, anxiety, and irritability and concluded that psychiatrists use these terms in a differentiated way; this is not however the case with most people and it is necessary to spend some time in the attempt to understand what the patient does mean by his statement. Argyle (1978) has pointed out the value of nonverbal communication in arriving at understanding of the patient's mental state; the slumped posture, hands twisting a handkerchief, tears standing in the eyes, or fingers drumming out on the chair arm some message of frustration or annoyance. Careful perception of such communication is often more valuable than detailed records of what was said. Allowance must also be made for differences in social class and background, ethnic origin, and education of the clinician and the patient; anxiety may be increased by the fact that the patient is in the unfamiliar territory of the general practitioner's consulting room or the hospital clinic and a large desk, covered with medical paraphernalia, between the patient and the clinician does nothing to increase confidence and the revelation of causes for distress.

The patient should be encouraged to talk about himself and his feelings, a procedure which is hindered by a list of questions, but most people need some help in knowing how to start to give relevant information whilst a few need gentle guidance to direct the flow of irrelevant information into more helpful channels. Sometimes a patient will expect his distress to be understood without the need for him to say much about himself, and the question 'Why do you think you feel as you do?' may initially cause some surprise; it is also a question avoided by some clinicians who think it may betray doubt and uncertainty on their part. However, an impression of certainty is best avoided until considerable knowledge has been acquired and the question is always revealing even when the answer is 'I honestly don't know'. Towards the end of the interview the clinician should tentatively formulate the situation and the resulting disorder of mood as he understands it, requesting comment and correction by some such phrase as 'Have I got it right?' He may bring the interview to a close by pointing out that mood disorders are everyday experiences that do not always require treatment apart from the opportunity to talk and to be understood; further comment should be invited and an early second appointment then offered.

Psychotherapy commences with the first encounter between the patient and the clinician. There is, of course, no stereotyped way of conducting an interview with a depressed person but if it is not carried out with sympathy and interest it is better not done at all; neither should a flesh wound be probed with an unsterilized instrument. If the clinician has insufficient time for an unpressed half-hour interview at the first contact it is better to admit this and to make an appointment for a later time. At the second interview the patient may be much better and his improvement may reasonably be attributed to the opportunity he has experienced to talk about his problem and situation to a professional person whose judgement he can respect so that he has been able to reflect upon his difficulty in the light of the clinician's reaction. The frequency of the occurrence of this improvement underlines the importance of not prescribing drugs at the first interview, for if this is done the improvement may be mistakenly attributed to the effect of the drug and medication may then be needlessly continued.

At the second interview the patient's situation is further explored on the basis of information already gained and towards the end of this session the nature of the depressive state will be clearer and a formulation of the condition with a plan of therapy may be made. Patients whose depressive state is essentially a grief reaction to loss or disappointment may not need much more help although some may require more time to work through their grief with the therapist. During this time he should be given the moral support and the encouragement to explore ways of adapting to his changed circumstances. His depression is to be considered as a normal reparative process and not as evidence of mental sickness or personal weakness.

The patient whose depression is clearly based upon negative self-concepts may require more intensive psychotherapeutic help, the form of which will depend on the particular training of the clinician but a relatively brief therapy which may produce lasting benefit after a few sessions is the process of cognitive restructuring of attitudes as outlined by Beck (1976). This therapy consists of exploring with the patient his misconceptions about himself and others and the resulting faulty conclusions that are habitually drawn. For instance, a patient may be in the habit of being gloomy and pessimistic for she has become convinced that her family and her neighbours do not like her; this may well be true but the situation has arisen because of her persistent withdrawal from every friendly advance in the past. She needs to be helped to experience the positive reaction of someone else to her own approach and should be encouraged to try this out in small ways with someone whom she does not know very well; a comment on the pretty dress the teenage assistant in the corner shop is wearing may be a suitable starting point. Gradually, and after some initial disappointments, she may learn that people can react with pleasure and interest to her comments and this process may gather force. Cognitive therapy is, of course, as old as history and finds expression in many proverbs and sayings such as 'Laugh and the world laughs with you'; the patient who is expecting the clinician to 'treat' her may be sceptical when informed that the procedure is a process of self-help. This attitude underlines Beck's expression of the necessity for 'therapeutic collaboration' which begins with the explanation that cognitive therapy is a tried method which depends for its success partly on the effort the patient is prepared to put into it and partly on the support and direction he will gain from the therapist; the collaboration, of course, consists of the patient's willingness to work for himself and with the therapist in bringing about change. Beck also draws attention to the paper of Orne and Wender (1968) that preliminary coaching of the patient in the principles of therapy appears to enhance its effectiveness.

The method of cognitive therapy must be applied with care to selected patients with the type of depressive neurosis outlined above. Its too liberal prescription for the multitude of patients suffering from mild but chronic depressive states may well do harm by increasing the despair experienced by some patients who feel that they are really incapable of making the effort directed by the therapist. Applied to the wrong patient, such a directive form of therapy may sometimes lead to a suicidal act. The patients for whom cognitive therapy is particularly contraindicated are those whose depression is based upon biological rather than psychological change. It is difficult to be certain about the presence of this form of depression but characteristics are its unvarying, all-pervasive nature, the central symptom of anhedonia in all situations, and a period of distinct change in the patient's outlook which occurred for no understandable reason. This form of depressive neurosis is therefore a mild form of the disorder most clinicians have no difficulty in recognizing in its more severe form as 'endogenous' depression. However, because of the relatively low level of the depressive symptomatology, the frequent admixture of neurotic symptoms such as phobias and irritability, and its tendency to chronicity, the label depressive neurosis often appears to be the most appropriate. If, after the initial period of assessment, it appears that the disorder is basically this variety of depression, then antidepressant drug therapy should be prescribed; in the case of doubt (and uncertainty about the outcome of drug therapy always exists) then antidepressants should usually be prescribed for a trial period for it is unlikely that any form of psychotherapy will be successful if an untreated biologically-based depressive state is the core of the disorder.

Certain rules must be followed in the matter of prescribing antidepressants. The patient must be told why such a drug is being prescribed, that there will certainly be a delay before its beneficial effects occur and that slightly uncomfortable side-effects will probably be experienced for a week or two before the benefit occurs. The patient should be given the opportunity to ask questions and express misgivings about drug treatment and he should certainly be assured that the drug is not a 'pep pill' to which he will become addicted. The toxic effect of the drugs when taken in overdosage should be kept in mind and large quantities should not be given to a potentially suicidal out-patient. A tricyclic antidepressant is probably the drug of first choice and treatment compliance will be increased if the drug selected is given as a single daily dose at night for in this way the patient is more likely to remember to take it, the maximum sedative effect, occurring some hours after ingestion, will relieve insomnia, and daytime side-effects will be lessened. Tricyclics have a long plasma half-life and there is no rationale for the conventional prescription of divided doses three or four times daily. Up to 150 mg can safely be given to a physically healthy adult at night but if a higher dose is required then the dose may be divided.

It is doubtful that any one tricyclic antidepressant has significant advantages over any other. It is usually believed that amitriptyline has greater sedative and anxiolytic effects than imipramine but this belief was based on assertion rather than experiment and a recent trial (Beaini, Hindmarch, and Snaith, 1980) has shown no difference between the two drugs. The chief reason for preferring one drug over another will be the form of its presentation; for instance one widely-prescribed tricyclic drug is presented as a 75 mg tablet and it will be more acceptable to the patient, requiring 225 mg, to take three tablets of this preparation than nine 25 mg tablets of another preparation. There is no advantage in the widespread practice of prescribing 'cocktails' of drugs and, in particular, the addition of the ubiquitous benzodiazepine sedatives to antidepressant regimes will only increase the degree of unacceptable drowsiness.

The dose of a tricyclic antidepressant should be increased to 200 mg daily, unless there is a clear response at a lower dosage when it may be maintained at that dose. Only if there is no response to this dose after a period of four to six weeks, should the depression be judged to be unresponsive to tricyclics and the trial of drug treatment abandoned. There is at present insufficient knowledge concerning response to other types of antidepressant drugs in the case where thorough treatment with tricyclics has failed, and rather than prolonging drug treatment in such patients consideration should be given to the indications of ECT; this treatment should not be withheld any longer from the patient who has the persisting features of a biologically-based depressive disorder as outlined earlier.

Although the therapy of depressive neurosis has been considered in sections according to the predominant type it may be restated that in practice combinations of types are common and a recognition of this will usually call for combinations of therapeutic techniques. Successful therapy may depend on the willingness of the therapist to review progress every few weeks and to change to a different plan or incorporate another technique into the programme if improvement appears to be unduly delayed. An excellent survey of the present state of knowledge concerning the treatment of depression has been carried out by Weissman (1979). She reviewed studies of cognitive therapy, behavioural therapy, interpersonal psychotherapy, group therapy, and marital therapy and concluded that combined treatment with antidepressant drugs and psychotherapy together produce the best results. However, she noted that some patients do not tolerate the drug treatment whilst others do not wish to enter into psychotherapy and she advised that, under either of these conditions, the patient should not be denied treatment but should be offered the alternative form. She concluded that data were still insufficient to say which of the psychotherapies should be used, which patients will recover quickly with no treatment or which subtype of depressive disorder will benefit from drugs and/or psychotherapy. She looked forward to the results of at least five studies which should be reported in the next three years and hoped that within the coming decade a scientifically supportable rationale for the treatment of the different types of depression would be available.

A NOTE ON IRRITABILITY

Irritability is a common disorder of mood but most textbooks of psychiatry make only a passing reference to it; compared with other mood disorders it ranks low in the amount of research attention it receives. Both anxiety neurosis and depressive neurosis have achieved established nosological status but the concept of an 'irritability neurosis' has not been proposed. In the Glossary to the 9th Revision of the *International classification of disease* irritability is mentioned as one of the symptoms of the now largely defunct category called neurasthenia, and the 9th Revision retains the concept of a type of personality disorder:

> 301.3 Explosive Personality Disorder. Personality disorder characterized by instability of mood with liability to intemperate outbursts of anger, hate, violence or affection. Aggression may be expressed in words or in physical violence. The outbursts cannot readily be controlled by the affected persons, who are not otherwise prone to antisocial behaviour.

The word irritability is used in a variety of senses and hostility, aggression, and anger are all involved in the concept. For the purpose of the present discussion irritability is defined as a state of poor control over aggressive impulses directed towards others and manifested verbally as shouting or snapping and physically by such acts as throwing objects, slamming doors, or directly assaulting others. It is also recognized that irritability may be directed more towards oneself than to others.

Irritability may be a trait of the personality structure, outbursts of bad temper being a permanent feature of the demeanour of the individual. Like other moods it may be provoked by certain circumstances, in which case it is considered to be a normal and understandable reaction. Irritability may also be the manifestation of a morbid disturbance of mood which is uncharacteristic of the individual's normal demeanour. It is this last form of irritability which will be discussed here. It is an age-dependent mood disorder the frequency and intensity of which decreases with age. Irritability is also more likely to be directed towards people who are in a close social relationship with the patient. This matter has been studied by Weissman and Paykel (1974) who have defined a 'continuum of intimacy' when irritability occurs in the context of a depressive illness in women; the expression of irritability is most pronounced towards the children, then the spouse, then members of the extended family and it is least pronounced towards workmates and friends outside the home. Weissman and Paykel note that assessment of irritability at, say, an out-patient clinic may give a very misleading impression of the intensity of the mood disorder when the patient is at home.

As with all mood disorders the formulation of the nature of irritability will depend upon a careful history and behavioural analysis. A guide to the intensity of the disorder relative to the other major mood disorders of depression and anxiety is readily obtained by the self-rated Irritability-Depression-Anxiety (IDA) Scale (Snaith *et al.*, 1978). This scale is a measure of the present state of the moods and, as such, provides a valid estimate of change over time or with treatment.

In women, irritability is frequently phasic when it forms a prominent component of the symptomatology of the premenstrual tension syndrome. The mood may occasionally be a symptom of organic brain disease and it may be a feature of chronic or acute alcoholic intoxication. It may also be precipitated by chronic ingestion of sedative drugs; irritability is a well-recognized unwanted effect of barbiturate drug therapy, especially when the drug is prescribed in the form of phenobarbitone for children with epilepsy; unfortunately this is often unrecognized by clinicians and the irritability is attributed to the epilepsy itself. Benzodiazepines may also cause the paradoxical effect (Ingram and Timbury, 1960) of precipitating marked irritability. The important matter of the relationship between the mood disorder and psychotropic drugs was discussed in a leading article of the *British Medical Journal* (1975).

Irritability may also be a prominent symptom in affective disorders and may overshadow the other disordered moods of depression and anxiety; an affective disorder should always be suspected when there is a clear account of a change in a patient's demeanour in which pronounced and persistent irritability occurs for no obvious reason.

Aggression (or hostility) plays a central role in the psychoanalytic theory of the genesis of depression; since the time of the writings of Freud and Abraham it has been held that depression is a result of hostility being introjected away from others towards the ego. However, this hypothesis has never been clearly substantiated and is in fact contradicted by the observation that marked irritability is a frequent symptom in some depressive states and moreover, when this is the case, the symptom tends to subside with recovery from the depression.

Two case histories will now be given to illustrate the differing psychopathological contexts in which irritability may occur.

> *Avril.* This married woman, aged 24, sought treatment for her fear of children; she wished to have a baby but could not trust herself to control her temper in the presence of children. This problem occurred in a wide context of intense irritability; for trivial or no sufficient reason she screamed and threw objects at her husband and, although she was fond of animals, she had once seized and killed her pet cat in a fit of ungovernable rage. The irritability had been a constant feature since adolescence; it was exacerbated by, but not confined to, the premenstrual period.
>
> Examination revealed a marked degree of pervasive anxiety in addition to the irritability; she was not depressed. She had previously received psychiatric treatment in which her symptoms had been interpreted in the light of the violent quarrels which occurred between her parents during her childhood. She and her husband had also attended a marriage guidance clinic for over a year. Neither of these interventions had helped her.

She followed the programme of anxiety control training (see Chapter 7) and after some weeks both the anxiety and the irritability began to diminish. After three months she became pregnant and this pregnancy was planned by both her husband and herself for they both felt that she was gaining better control over her abnormal moods. She continued with the programme throughout her pregnancy and the postnatal period and when she was interviewed two years after the birth she had formed normal affectional bonds to the child, had no fear of handling him, and the husband confirmed that tranquillity was now the keynote in the domestic scene.

Harry B. This married man, aged 40, was referred on account of a depressive state which had persisted for a year. There was no major precipitant or circumstance to account for the disorder of mood. At examination the most prominent symptom was irritability and he admitted that his daughter could not tolerate his abusive language and had left home and that he had been barred from membership of a club on account of his offensive behaviour. Depressive symptomatology was also present. His wife confirmed that previous to the onset of his illness his family and social relationships had been harmonious and that everyone was perplexed and alarmed by the change in his demeanour.

Treatment with imipramine was commenced and within six weeks both irritability and depressive symptoms had been completely relieved.

So far as drug therapy for irritability is concerned, tricyclic antidepressant drugs should be prescribed when the symptom occurs in the setting of an affective illness; even when this is not clearly the case a trial of the drug may sometimes produce beneficial results. Benzodiazepine and other sedative drugs should on no account be prescribed for a person prone to irritability; there is a real possibility of converting a potential into an actual 'batterer'. Lithium carbonate has gained a slight reputation for an 'antiaggressive' effect (Sheard *et al*, 1976; Worrall, Moody and Naylor, 1975); this is an interesting observation which has so far received little attention.

References

AKISKAL, H. S. and McKINNEY, W. T. (1975). Overview of recent research in depression. *Archs gen. Psychiat.* **32**, 285–305.
—— BITAR, A. H., PUZANTIAN, V. R., ROSENTHAL, T. L., and WALKER, P. W. (1978). The nosological status of neurotic depression. *Archs gen. Psychiat.* **35**, 756–66.
ALARCON, R. D. and COVI, L. (1972). The precipitating event in depression. *J. nerv. ment. Dis.* **155**, 379–91.
ANDREWS, G. and TENNANT, C. (1978). Life event stress and psychiatric illness. *Psychol. Med.* **8**, 545–9.

ARGYLE, M. (1978). Non-verbal communication and mental disorder. *Psychol. Med.* **8**, 551–4.

*ASCHER, E. (1952). A criticism of the concept of neurotic depression. *Am. J. Psychiat.* **108**, 901–8.

BEAINI, A. Y., HINDMARCH, I., and SNAITH, R. P. (1980). A re-examination of the clinical effects of imipramine and amitriptyline in depressive illness. *J. affect. Disord.* **2**, 89–94.

BECK, A. T. (1967). *Depression; clinical, experimental and theoretical aspects.* Staples Press, London.

—— (1976). *Cognitive therapy and the emotional disorders.* International Universities Press, New York.

British Medical Journal (1975). Tranquillizers causing aggression. Leading article. *Br. med. J.* **i**, 113–14.

BROWN, F. (1966). Childhood bereavement and subsequent psychiatric disorder. *Br. J. Psychiat.* **112**, 1035–41.

BROWN, G. W. and HARRIS, T. (1978). Social origins of depression: a reply. *Psychol. Med.* **8**, 577–88.

CADIE, M., NYE, F J., and STOREY, P. (1976). Anxiety and depression after infectious mononucleosis. *Br. J. Psychiat.* **128**, 559–61.

CLAYTON, P. J., DESMARAIS, L., and WINOKUR, G. (1968). A study of normal bereavement. *Am. J. Psychiat.* **125**, 168–78.

—— HALIKAS, J. A., and MAURICE, W. L. (1972). The depression of widowhood. *Br. J. Psychiat.* **120**, 71–8.

CYTRYN, L. and McKNEW, D. H. (1972). Proposed classification of childhood depression. *Am. J. Psychiat.* **129**, 149–55.

DALTON, K. (1971). Prospective study into puerperal depression. *Br. J. Psychiat.* **118**, 689–92.

DENNEHY, C. M. (1966). Childhood bereavement and psychiatric illness. *Br. J. Psychiat.* **112**, 1049–69.

FOULDS, G. A. (1973). The relationship between the depressive illnesses. *Br. J. Psychiat.* **123**, 531–3.

FREUD, S. (1917). Mourning and melancholia. In *Collected papers*, Vol. 4 (ed. E. Jones). Hogarth Press and the Institute of Psychoanalysis, London.

FROMMER, E. A. (1968). Depression in childhood. In *Recent developments in affective disorders* (ed. A. Coppen and A. Walk). *British Journal of Psychiatry*, Special Publication, Number 2. Headley Bros, Ashford.

GILLESPIE. R. D. (1929). The clinical differentiation of types of depression. *Guy's Hosp. Rep.* **79**, 306–44.

GRAHAM, P. (1974). Depression in prepubertal children. *Devl Med. child Neurol.* **16**, 340–9.

GRANVILLE-GROSSMAN, K. L. (1968). The early environment in affective disorder. In *Recent developments in affective disorders* (ed. A. Coppen and A. Walk). *British Journal of Psychiatry*, Special Publication, Number 2. Headley Brothers, Ashford.

HAMILTON, M. and WHITE, J. M. (1959). Clinical syndromes in depressive states. *J. ment. Sci.* **105**, 985–98.

HAYS, P. (1964). Modes of onset of psychotic depression. *Br. med. J.* **ii**, 779–84.

HUDGENS, R. W., MORRISON, J. R., and BARCHHA, R. D. (1967). Life events and the onset of primary affective disorders. *Archs gen. Psychiat.* **16**, 134–45.

INGRAM, I. M. and TIMBURY, G. C. (1960). The side-effects of Librium. *Lancet* **ii**, 766.

KENDELL, R. E. (1969). The continuum mode of depressive illness. *Proc. R. Soc. Med.* **62**, 335–9.

*—— (1976). The classification of depression: a review. *Br. J. Psychiat.* **129**, 15–28.

—— WAINWRIGHT, S., HAILEY, A., and SHANNON, B. (1976). The influence of childbirth on psychiatric morbidity. *Psychol. Med.* **6**, 297–302.

KERR, T. A., SCHAPIRA, A., and ROTH, M. (1969). The relationship between premature death and affective disorders. *Br. J. Psychiat.* **115**, 1277–82.

KILOH, L. G., ANDREWS, G., NEILSON, M., and BIANCHI, G. N. (1972). The relationship of the syndromes called endogenous and neurotic depression. *Br. J. Psychiat.* **121**, 183–96.

KLEIN, M. (1948). Contributions to the psychogenesis of manic-depressive states. In *Contributions to psychoanalysis, 1921–1945.* Hogarth Press, London.

KLERMAN, G. L., ENDICOTT, J., SPITZER, R., and HIRSCH-FIELD, R. M. A. (1979). Neurotic depressions: a systematic analysis of multiple criteria and meanings. *Am. J. Psychiat.* **136**, 57–61.

*KOLVIN, I. and NICOL, A. R. (1979). Child psychiatry. In *Recent advances in clinical psychiatry*, Vol. 3 (ed. K. Granville-Grossman). Churchill Livingstone, Edinburgh.

LAZARUS, A. A. (1968). Learning theory and the treatment of depression. *Behav. Res. Ther.* **6**, 83–9.

LEFF, J. P. (1978). Psychiatrists' versus patients' concepts of unpleasant emotions. *Br. J. Psychiat.* **133**, 306–13.

LESSE, S. (1968). The multivariant masks of depression. *Am. J. Psychiat.* **124** (May Suppl.), 35–40.

*LEWIS, A. (1934). Melancholia: a clinical survey of depressive states. *J. ment. Sci.* **80**, 277–378.

—— (1938). States of depression; their clinical and aetiological differentiation. *Br. med. J.* **ii**, 875–8.

LIBERMAN, R. P. and RASKIN, D. E. (1971). Depression: a behavioural formulation. *Archs gen. Psychiat.* **24**, 515–23.

*McAULEY, R. (1979). Behaviour therapy and depression: a review of some aspects of aetiology and treatment. In *Current themes in psychiatry* (ed. R. N. Gaind and B. L. Hudson). Macmillan, London.

MAPOTHER, E. (1926). Discussion on manic-depressive psychosis. *Br. med. J.* **ii**, 877–9.

*MENDELS, J. and COCHRANE, C. (1968). The nosology of depression: the endogenous–reactive concept. *Am. J. Psychiat.* **124** (May Suppl.), 1–11.

MEYER, A. (1905). Discussant in The classification of melancholias. *J. nerv. ment. Dis.* **32**, 112–17.

MUNRO, A. (1966). Some familial and social factors in depressive illness. *Br. J. Psychiat.* **112**, 429–41.

ORNE, M. T. and WENDER, P. H. (1968). Anticipatory socialization for psychotherapy: method and rationale. *Am. J. Psychiat.* **124**, 1202–12.

PAYKEL, E. S. (1971). Classification of depressed patients: a cluster analysis. *Br. J. Psychiat.* **118**, 275–88.

—— MYERS, J. K., DIENELT, M. N., KLERMAN, G. L., LINDEN-THAL, J. J., and PEPPER, M. P. (1969). Life events and depression: a controlled study. *Archs gen. Psychiat.* **21**, 753–60.

*PITT, B. (1968). 'Atypical' depression following childbirth. *Br. J. Psychiat.* **114**, 1325–35.

POLLITT, J. (1977). Sex difference and the mind. *Proc. R. Soc. Med.* **70**, 145–8.

SELIGMAN, M. E. P. (1975). Helplessness. In *Depression, development and death*. Freeman, San Francisco, California.

SIMS, A. (1978). Hypotheses linking neuroses with premature mortality. *Psychol. Med.* **8**, 255–63.

SHEARD, M. H., MARINI, J. L., BRIDGES, C. I., and WAGNER, E. (1976). The effect of lithium on impulsive, aggressive behaviour in man. *Am. J. Psychiat.* **133**, 1409–13.

SLATER, E. and ROTH, M. (1969). *Clinical psychiatry*. Ballière, Tindall and Cassell, London.

SNAITH, R. P., CONSTANTOPOULOS, A. A., JARDINE, M. Y., and McGUFFIN, P. (1978). A clinical scale for the self-assessment of irritability. *Br. J. Psychiat.* **132**, 164–71.

SPICER, C. C., HARE, E. H., and SLATER, E. (1973). Neurotic and psychotic forms of depressive illness: evidence from age influence. *Br. J. Psychiat.* **123**, 535–41.

STENSTEDT, A. (1966). The genetics of neurotic depression. *Acta psychiat. scand.* **42**, 392–409.

*TENNANT, C. and ANDREWS, G. (1978). The cause of life events in neurosis. *J. Psychosom. Res.* **22**, 41–5.

*TYRER, P. (1976). Towards rational therapy with monoamine oxidase inhibitors. *Br. J. Psychiat.* **128**, 354–60.

*WEISSMAN, M. M. (1979). The psychological treatment of depression: evidence for the efficacy of psychotherapy alone, in comparison with, and in combination with pharmacotherapy. *Archs gen. Psychiat.* **36**, 1261–9.

—— and KLERMAN, G. L. (1977). Sex differences and the epidemiology of depression. *Archs gen. Psychiat.* **34**, 98–111.

—— and PAYKEL, E. S. (1974). *The depressed woman, a study of social relationships*. University of Chicago Press, Illinois.

WELNER, Z. (1978). Childhood depression: an overview. *J. nerv. ment. Dis.* **166**, 588–93.

WEST, E. D. and DALLY, P. J. (1959). The effects of iproniazid in depressive syndromes. *Br. med. J.* **i**, 1491–4.

WORLD HEALTH ORGANIZATION (1978). *Mental disorders: glossary* and guide to their classification in accordance with the 9th Revision of the International Classification of Diseases. Geneva.

WORRALL, E. P., MOODY, J. P., and NAYLOR, G. J. (1975). Lithium in nonmanic-depressives: antiaggressive effect and red blood cell lithium values. *Br. J. Psychiat.* **126**, 464–8.

3

Obsessional neurosis

CONCEPTS AND DEFINITIONS

SINCE the time that Esquirol first described a case and Morel first used the term obsession (Black, 1974), obsessional neurosis has been subject to frequent redefinition. Three types of phenomena are included in the concept:

1. Long periods of brooding thought which may be concerned with some potential calamity or some unanswerable question.
2. Impulses to act in an aggressive or socially offensive manner. The impulse may not be carried into action but remain as a thought with a 'what if I should?' quality, e.g. uttering blasphemies in church or stabbing a child with a knife; or the impulse may be carried out as, for example, in some cases of genital exhibitionism.
3. Engagement in prolonged, iterative behaviour such as counting, checking, washing, or cleaning to an inordinate degree.

Obsessional thoughts are usually called ruminations whereas actions are frequently referred to as compulsions; however the use of the latter term is a source of confusion for many definitions state that compulsiveness is a feature of all obsessional phenomena; it is therefore proposed that the term rumination should be retained for obsessional thinking but that actions should be referred to as obsessional rituals if they are prolonged and iterative, or as obsessional impulses if they are brief and not repeated in a single session. The frequently used adjectival term 'obsessive-compulsive' contains a redundant element and the syndrome will be referred to as obsessional neurosis. A special mention must be made of obsessional fears and their differentiation from phobias, for this is also a source of confusion and some authors do not distinguish between the phenomena; Marks (1969) has clarified the point: 'An obsessional fear is not a direct fear of a given object or situation but rather of the imagined consequences arising therefrom.' Thus, a person with a phobia of dogs will experience extreme anxiety at the sight of a dog whereas the person with an obsessional fear will not experience so much anxiety at the sight of the dog but will engage in prolonged anxious concern in case he has been contaminated by the dog and it is likely that he will worry more about dogs that he does not see than those that he does.

It is important to realize that the three types of phenomena are not usually independent of each other (if they were, their combined inclusion under the rubric of obsessional neurosis would not be possible); for instance obsessional rituals of cleaning occur in response to ruminations concerning contamination and an obsessional counting ritual may be a device for holding an obsessional impulse under control. In an Indian study (Akhtar *et al.*, 1975) the authors distinguished between the *content* and the *form* of an obsession, giving clear examples and definitions; *forms* were classified as doubts, thinking, fears, images, impulses, and actions (which they called 'compulsions'). The *content* of an obsession may be concerned, for instance, with aggressive themes, contamination, security, or metaphysical speculations. However in the course of time both content and form may alter and recombine in a single case, as is illustrated by the following history:

Mary was a 25-year-old married woman who had not suffered from psychiatric disorder until the late stage of her second pregnancy three years previously. The first obsessional ruminations were concerned with possible harm to the foetus. After the child was born she continued to fear that she would harm the child and she developed an overmeticulous regime of sterilizing all utensils which might come into contact with the child; she spent about three hours a day in activity such as boiling spoons and reboiling them if the thought occurred that she might have accidentally touched one whilst not wearing her sterilized rubber gloves. When the child was a few months old the thought first occurred to her that she might strangle the child and this thought increased in frequency until it occluded the concern of harm by default so that she spent a large part of the day searching for cords, belts, string, and so forth, removing them from the house and burning them.

The definition of an obsessional phenomenon has centred around the themes of a subjective sense of compulsion, a resistance to carrying it out, and a recognition by the individual of its senseless nature. Schneider (1925) emphasized the first and last of these elements in his definition:

> Contents of consciousness which are accompanied by the experience of subjective compulsion and which cannot be got rid of, though on quiet reflection they are recognized as senseless.

Lewis (1936) stated that the essential feature of an obsession was the subjective sense of compulsion from which the other features followed. Twenty-one years later he again recognized the primacy of the sense of compulsion against which the patient engaged in a fruitless struggle with an experience which he recognized as alien to himself:

> Along with this subjective feeling of compulsion goes an inability to accept the experience as part of one's proper integrated mental activity: it is a foreign body, not implanted from without (as a disordered schizophrenic experience might be held to be by the patient) but arising from within, home-made but disowned, a sort of mental sequestrum, a calculus that keeps on causing trouble (Lewis, 1957).

Kraüpl Taylor (1966) has pointed out that the psychotic patient may be said to be 'obsessively' preoccupied with a delusional idea but that such a preoccupation could not be considered to be an obsessional symptom. He traced the distinction back to demonological theories and the distinction between *possession* and *obsession*; in the latter, the evil spirits surround the individual (Latin: *obsidere*, to besiege) whereas in possession the spirit enters into its victim and dominates him completely. If the phrase 'morbid ideation' is substituted for evil spirits and if we leave the realm of demonology for that of psychopathology, then the distinction between a neurotic and a psychotic symptom revolves around the familiar theme of the retention of insight into the morbid nature of the idea.

More recent work has again challenged any undue tendency for the encapsulation of what is to be considered as essential to the definition of an obsessional symptom. Walker (1973) has argued that resistance is neither a sufficient nor a necessary condition for a thought or action to be defined as obsessional and she gives examples of patients in whom the sense of compulsion was present but the resistance to the compulsion was absent. Stern and Cobb (1978) carried out an analysis of the attitudes of adult patients suffering from obsessional neurosis and their families towards the symptoms;

possible sources of bias in their sample were that all the patients carried out some form of behavioural response to an obsessional thought and the patients had been referred for therapy on account of subjective distress or distress to the family. Of their sample, 78 per cent of the patients considered their rituals to be silly or absurd and only 54 per cent showed more than a slight resistance to carrying out the ritual. The authors concluded that Schneider's criterion of the 'recognition of the senselessness' of the obsessional symptom was a more important element than a resistance to it and they offered a revised definition:

> The obsessive-compulsive neurosis consists of either ruminations (or ideas) which are psychic phenomena recurring in spite of the patient regarding them as alien and absurd and/or voluntary motor actions which are reluctantly performed despite their being regarded as alien or absurd.

Lewis (1936) warned of the danger of classifying as obsessions all kinds of repetitive behaviour, especially those acts with a forensic implication such as sexual offences. He considered that the labelling of some forms of antisocial behaviour as psychiatric disorder could only lead to a confusion of the psychiatrist's proper sphere of activity. Nevertheless, it is necessary to examine some types of disordered behaviour and to consider whether sometimes such behaviour may be considered to be obsessional. A good example is that of gambling which, when carried out to excess, is sometimes loosely referred to as compulsive gambling. Moran (1970) rejected this term and concluded that the phenomenon of pathological gambling could be classified under the broad categories of (a) subcultural gambling, (b) neurotic gambling, (c) impulsive gambling, (d) psychopathic gambling, and (e) symptomatic gambling. The impulsive variety is associated with a loss of control and ambivalence to the activity, so that whilst being longed for it is also dreaded, since it has become irresistible; a literary example of this variety is provided by the grandfather in Dickens's *Old curiosity shop*, whose irresistible urge led him into degrading associations but who always hoped that a final win would compensate for his long and unbroken series of losses. Neither Dickens's character nor Dostoevsky who, himself a pathological gambler, described his own passion and affliction in *The gambler*, could be said to suffer from an obsessional symptom in the terms set out in this chapter; they may have been acting under a drive of compulsive strength but there was also an eager anticipation of the act which is certainly lacking in the obsessional neurotic engaging upon his ritual. However, in Moran's fifth category gambling may be symptomatic of a mental illness, most commonly depression, and in such instances the behaviour may have the hallmarks of a true obsessional symptom being regarded by the patient as senseless, not enjoyed, resisted yet always succumbed to under the influence of the overpowering compulsion. In like manner there are occasions when impulsive acts of theft, often of trivial and unneeded articles, are committed by depressed patients and these also may sometimes have the characteristics of obsessional impulses.

Exhibitionism provides a further example to illustrate the debate. Genital display is certainly not symptomatic of a single homogeneous psychopathological entity; in his survey of the literature Rooth (1971) concluded that descriptions of exhibitionism fell into two main categories. In the first, the individual is an inhibited young man who struggles against the impulse to expose but finds it irresistible; he displays a flaccid penis, derives no erotic gratification or other pleasure from the act, and feels humiliated by his strange behaviour. The second type is the obverse picture; he masturbates during exposure, shows little shame, and manifests a number of other sociopathic traits. Rickles (1942) is also of the opinion that there are a number of causes for the behaviour but that one variety is a form of obsessional neurosis and a recent case history supports this view:

> David, a married man of 23, was referred for a psychiatric report; he was charged with the offence of indecent exposure and had previously appeared before a court on the same charge. He did not manifest other sociopathic symptoms, his sexual orientation was heterosexual and the marital relationship was harmonious both in the sexual and general respect. He first exposed at the age of 11 years and had continued to do so at irregular intervals since; on no occasion was the behaviour motivated by erotic excitement and he had never derived pleasure from the act. He did not wish to frighten or alarm his 'victim' but required that some sort of notice should be taken of the act; he felt anxious when about to expose but calmer afterwards. He felt compelled to expose and knew that resistance on his part was useless; he considered the behaviour was humiliating and inexplicable and was strongly motivated to cooperate in treatment.

This man suffered from a deviance of behaviour with the hallmarks of an obsessional impulse.

NATURE AND CAUSES

It is sometimes considered that obsessional neurosis is the most circumscribed of the neurotic syndromes but this view cannot be upheld and obsessional symptoms may occur in the context of many forms of mental disorder. This fact has been recognized by most theorists who have attempted to consider the genesis of the symptoms rather than explain the nature of the psychopathological entity termed obsessional neurosis; however, Freud and the early psychoanalysts were more sanguine in their views of all-encompassing explanations of the phenomena and of the neurosis.

Psychoanalytic views

Early in his writings, Freud (1896) included obsessional neurosis with the neuropsychoses of defence based on the concept that the symptoms 'arose through the psychical mechanism of (unconscious) defence — that is, an attempt to repress an incompatible idea which had come into distressing opposition to the patient's ego.' At this stage he admitted that he could not give a definite account of the aetiology of obsessional neurosis but he put forward the view that the repressed experiences were of a sexual nature; in contradistinction to hysteria, where these were of a passive nature, in obsessional neurosis the trauma had an aggressive slant and this accounted for his belief that the disorder was more common in men. According to this view, obsessional symptoms are transformed self-reproaches for some sexual act performed in childhood; such events, which contain the germ of the later neurosis, are acts of sexual aggression towards the opposite sex and these are repressed to be replaced by the primary symptoms of defence such as conscientiousness, shame, and self-reproach. The emergence of the illness is considered to be characterized by a failure of defence and a return of the repressed memories which re-emerge into consciousness in an altered form; although the content of the symptom is now non-sexual it was supposed that it could be traced to the sexual act by a logical train of thought. The ego then seeks to fend off this acknowledgement and, in the struggle, creates the secondary defence symptoms such as ritual acts which, in the attempt to dam back the unwelcome memories, now assume as contrary a character as possible, rituals being concerned with purification and ruminations with such suprasensual matters as religious themes; or else the patient tries to master his memories by a recourse to testing and doubting things.

The next major development in psychoanalytic thinking about the nature of obsessional neurosis was that of regression to the pregenital anal-erotic stage of development. This development has been summarized by Fenichel (1945) who wrote that:

> Overt or concealed tendencies towards cruelty, or reaction formations against them are constant findings in compulsion neuroses.... This constant association of traits of cruelty and of anal eroticism in compulsion neuroses, to which Jones first drew attention, was what convinced Freud of the close relationship of the two types of phenomena, and of the existence of an 'anal-sadistic' stage of libido organization. In hysteria the repressed ideas remain unaltered in the unconscious and continue to exert their influence, from there. In so far as the Oedipus complex is the basis of compulsive symptoms, too, this also holds true for compulsion neurosis; but here, in addition to the Oedipus complex, very strong anal and sadistic impulses, which originated in the preceding period, regularly are operative and combated.... Compulsion neurotics are generally and obviously concerned about conflicts between aggressiveness and submissiveness, cruelty and gentleness, dirtiness and cleanliness, disorder and order.

He then went on to divide obsessional neurosis into two types, acute and chronic. In the former, anal sadistic regression occurred in childhood which rendered the individual liable to the neurotic reaction in later life. In the more frequent chronic neurosis:

> The sexuality that emerges at puberty takes a course analogous to that pursued by the sexuality of early childhood, and another regression to the anal-sadistic level takes place. The superego, with whose protests the new wave of anal-sadistic sexual wishes now comes into conflict, is itself unable to escape the effects of regression. It has become more sadistic and rages against the anal and sadistic instinctual demands not less than previously against the genital ones. It rages equally relentlessly against the offshoots of the phallic Oedipus wishes proper, which have persisted along with the anal-sadistic drives.... The continuous struggle on two fronts and the adjustments the ego makes to the symptoms (secondary defensive conflicts, counter-compulsions against compulsive symptoms, further reactions formations, the tendency of the symptoms to evolve from defence to gratification) complicate the subsequent development.

Reasoning such as this, once referred to by the American physician Weir Mitchell as 'these German perplexities' (quoted by Veith,

1965) did not however fully satisfy even their authors and in his study *Inhibitions, symptoms and anxiety* Freud (1926) wrote: 'it must be confessed that, if we endeavour to penetrate more deeply into its nature [of the obsessional neurosis] we still have to rely upon doubtful assumptions and unconfirmed suppositions.'

The contribution of learning theory

The attempt to explain the phenomena of obsessional neurosis from the standpoint of learning theory has run into insuperable difficulties and no major progress has been made. In their early enthusiasm to explain most types of neurotic symptoms in terms of this model, Eysenck and Rachman (1965) quoted experiments on animals, such as those conducted by Maier, who confronted rats with insoluble discrimination problems and noted that they developed stereotyped and rigid jumping responses when forced to move by electric shocks or a blast of air; these responses were referred to as 'fixations' and it was noted that they might persist when the noxious stimulus was withdrawn. Eysenck and Rachman then refer to the 'fixations' as 'compulsions' and take the unwarranted step of implying that obsessional symptoms in human beings have been, at least partly, explained by such experiments.

Wolpe (1958) considered that there were two types of phenomena which he termed 'anxiety-reducing' obsessions and 'anxiety-elevating' obsessions. In the former type the behaviour is considered to be a reaction to anxiety which it serves to reduce, at least for a short period of time, but in some cases a secondary increase in anxiety occurs following the initial reduction; for example obsessional eating may at first reduce anxiety and this may be followed by renewed anxiety at the thought of becoming fat. It is also considered that earlier in the lives of the patients some real threat was consistently dealt with by a well-defined behavioural response which then reappears during periods of stress and anxiety later in life. Wolpe relates as an example, the story of a girl whose father despised women; she found that she could counteract her father's blatant hostility by intellectual achievement and in consequence 'thinking things out' became her stereotyped response to anxiety. When, in later life, she developed an anxiety state she resorted to this problem-solving behaviour but when the anxiety could not be reduced by solving well-defined problems she set herself ever more complex problems such as the reason why people were good or bad. Wolpe paid less attention to attempting to explain anxiety-elevating obsessions and confined himself to quoting the case history of a man who suffered from a terrifying thought that he might strike people. Years previously he had been punished for reasons which he considered to be unjust and he had struck a military policeman; horror at the implications of this act increased the disturbance of his state of mind. Eleven years later, on arriving home to find his house crowded with his wife's relatives, he became violent, the police were called and he was again sent to jail; after his release, and still burning with a sense of injustice, he felt an impulse to strike a man who was offering him a lift in his car and he again felt the impulse when he again saw his wife; following this, he experienced the impulse to strike people in a variety of situations and he felt anxious at the sight of potentially dangerous implements such as knives.

Teasdale (1974) has examined the hypotheses of the nature of obsessional symptoms which have been derived from experimental studies of animal and human learning. The long-held view that an obsessional ritual is a form of avoidance response to a supposed noxious stimulus is difficult to uphold since an increase in anxiety frequently accompanies and follows the performance of the ritual (Walker and Beech, 1969). Teasdale considers that the avoidance-avoidance conflict paradigm is a more profitable explanation; according to this model the individual must make a choice between two responses, both of which are negatively reinforced, i.e. both performance and non-performance of the ritual have aversive consequences; moreover, it is probable that the conflict involved in the avoidance-avoidance situation serves further to increase the likelihood of an oscillation between the alternative responses and this could be considered to be the source of the doubt and uncertainty as to whether or not the ritual should be performed. This model may provide some explanation of the behaviour of the obsessional patient displaying certain types of symptoms but it does not offer an explanation as to why the aversive circumstance, such as fears of contamination, first occurs to such a morbid degree. It is possible that early experiences and particular traits of personality may play a role in some cases.

The difficulties which beset explanations of this type increase many times when the obsessional phenomenon is not a motor response to an anxious thought but simply the repetitive intrusion into consciousness of an anxious thought or impulse alone. As Meyer and Chesser (1970) wrote:

> The handwashing ritual is secondary to the idea of being contaminated and it is only these secondary symptoms which appear to be anxiety reducing responses. The origin of the obsessional idea of contamination (the primary symptom) still has to be accounted for. . . . Internal stimuli of which the patient is unaware may be functioning as conditioned fear stimuli. Whether or not this is so there is some controversy about the role of unconscious conditioned stimulus generalization, the prominence of the ideational component, its repetitiveness and persistence, remain the important feature to be accounted for.

Disorder of mood and the genesis of obsessions

The relationship of obsessional symptoms to depressive illness has been recognized for many years. In his careful study of the clinical features of melancholia, Lewis (1934) observed that 13 of the 61 patients manifested obsessional symptoms during the course of the illness and he noted that Henry Maudsley had subscribed to the view that obsessional disorder was a variety of affective illness. Stengel (1945) considered that cyclical depressive illness could present with such prominent obsessional symptoms that the underlying nature of the illness was frequently overlooked; he considered that these cases of obsessions, arising on the basis of depressive illness, accounted for those records of 'obsessional neurosis' that took a periodic course.

In a series of papers, Gittleson (1966) undertook a retrospective analysis of patients suffering from depressive psychosis who had been admitted to the Maudsley Hospital. The significance of his findings are unfortunately obscured by the inclusion of suicidal ruminations under the heading of obsessional symptoms but, even when these are excluded, over 25 per cent of patients suffered from obsessions during the depressive illness. Some patients who suffered from obsessional symptoms before the onset of the depression apparently lost the symptom during the course of the depression but this observation may have simply been due to their being overshadowed by the more severe symptoms of the psychosis. Of those patients who had suffered from obsessions before the depression some 14 per cent experienced a worsening of the original symptom after recovery from the depression, an effect which the author (quoting Anderson) referred to as 'a turn of the obsessional screw'.

There is no clear information in Gittleson's study as to the proportion of patients who, developing an obsessional symptom for the first time during the key depressive illness, also retained the symptom following recovery from the illness. However, examination of the data suggests that about 3 per cent did so; it is of interest to consider the possibility that a proportion of those patients, recorded as having obsessions before the key illness, may have first developed their enduring symptom during an earlier depressive episode. It is therefore possible that a number of patients suffering from obsessional neurosis or obsessional symptoms first developed such a disorder during a period of affective disorder. Some authors have emphasized the aggressive content of obsessions occurring during a depressive illness but Gittleson, while noting that aggressive themes such as harming people with knives, frequently emerged during the depression, they still accounted for less than half of all obsessional symptoms during the illness, suicidal ruminations excluded.

The relationship between obsessional neurosis and affective disorder has also been investigated from the vantage point of family history studies. Brown (1942) found that 8 per cent of the parents and 2 per cent of the siblings of obsessional neurotics suffered from manic-depressive psychosis, these figures being higher than for the other diagnostic categories of anxiety neurosis and hysteria and for the controls. Rüdin (1953) found that, among 130 obsessional propositi, the incidence of manic-depressive psychosis among uncles, aunts, grandparents, and parents was higher than in the general population although it was not higher among the siblings, possibly because many had not yet reached the peak age of risk for the occurrence of the psychosis. Black (1974) has summarized the genetic studies of obsessional neurosis and it is clear that, although there may be a hereditary element in the aetiology, this operates through the factors of personality structure and vulnerability to other forms of psychiatric disorder.

The relationship of obsessional symptoms to an underlying disorder of mood has been examined in a series of papers by Beech and his colleagues. In one paper (Beech, 1971) the author noted that an underlying mood disorder appeared to be the primary event in a chain culminating in obsessional behaviour and that the mood was characterized by depression and irritability rather than by anxiety. The view was put forward that, although attempts to 'disconnect' obsessional behaviour from specific cues may lead to temporary success, the continuing vulnerability of the patient's arousal system rapidly led to recurrence of obsessional symptoms of a similar or of a different kind. An example of the genesis of an obsessional symptom in association with a mood disorder is recorded by Beech and Perigault (1974):

> A patient had suffered from increasing disorder of mood for a period of some weeks. One morning, whilst on his motorcycle, he had to swerve in order to avoid an accident. From that moment the idea that he might unintentionally kill someone became insistent and irresistible and, from that time, it became necessary for him to check that such an accident had not occurred and, later, to check that the mere possibility of such an accident should not arise.

In an earlier paper, Walker and Beech (1969) made careful observations of three patients suffering from obsessional neurosis and, from these observations, they challenged many of the established views concerning the nature of the disorder. The observations were:

1. That irritability, depression and anxiety are all important components of the mood state associated with ritualistic behaviour;
2. These three components vary together;
3. That long rituals are associated with bad mood states and that the mood may worsen as the ritual continues;
4. That artificial curtailment of rituals has a beneficial effect on mood.

The last of these observations was contrary to the long-held belief that the obsessional ritual was an anxiety-relieving device and that its interruption was undertaken at peril of a further deterioration of the patient's condition.

Makhlouf-Norris and Norris (1973) studied obsessional neurosis using Kelly's repertory grid technique and discussed their findings in terms of the hypothesis that obsessions are devices which serve to reduce uncertainty of the individual about himself. Millar (1980) in a further investigation of the problem did not replicate Makhlouf-Norris and Norris's finding that obsessionals were differentiated by a particular type of cognitive structure; the obsessional group in Millar's study, although not showing sustained depression of mood, was clearly differentiated from normals and from other neurotics by a very negative, isolated, and extreme view of the self. Such a negative cognitive set is similar to that associated with depressive states, and the author notes that this finding is consistent with the view that the obsessional symptom is a coping device which defends against the occurrence of a depression which might otherwise be expected to occur. This view is of interest, but, if correct, it is probable that the obsession is, at best, only partially successful in fending off the mood change and, since most obsessional patients do experience permanent or recurrent depression of mood the obsessional symptom is a mental mechanism which attempts to 'make sense' of the otherwise subjectively and objectively inexplicable mental disorder.

The role of personality in the genesis of obsessions

It is usually considered that some special traits of personality must be present and are a necessary factor for the establishment of an obsessional neurosis and some authors have considered that the neurosis is nothing more than an exaggeration of underlying premorbid traits. There has, however, been no complete agreement on the features of this personality structure and a rather vague picture emerges.

Freud's (1908) description of anal erotism became enshrined in psychoanalytic thinking on the subject and the editors of the standard edition of his works, in the preface to the paper, comment:

> The theme of this paper has now become so familiar that it is difficult to realize the astonishment and indignation which it aroused on its first publication. The three character traits which are here associated with anal erotism (orderliness, parsimony and obstinacy) had, as we learn from Ernest Jones, already been mentioned by Freud in a letter to Jung of October 27th, 1906. He had associated money and miserliness with faeces in a letter to Fliess of December 22nd, 1897. The paper was no doubt partly stimulated by the analysis of the 'Rat Man' (1909), which had been concluded shortly before, though the specific connection between anal erotism and obsessional neurosis was only brought out some years later, in The Disposition To Obsessional Neurosis (1913). Another case history, that of the 'Wolf Man' (1918) led to a further expansion of the topic.

The word anankastic (Greek, *anankasmos*, compulsion) has been applied to both the symptom and the personality type and in the latter sense refers to traits of rigidity, conscientiousness, reliability, punctuality, and moral scrupulousness (Leigh, Pare, and Marks, 1977). In his examination of a series of patients suffering from obsessional neurosis, Pollitt (1960) found that a third had shown no obsessional traits in their premorbid personality and that 'anankasts' were more liable to fall ill with a depression than an obsessional neurosis. Lewis (1936) was doubtful that any particular personality type underlay the neurosis but he considered that two main personality patterns were found in obsessional neurotics *who had shown symptoms since childhood*: the first was obstinate, morose, and irritable and the other vacillating, lacking in self-confidence, and submissive. However, he was uncertain as to whether the supposed personality traits of patients were not in fact symptoms of their illness and it has been noted that he was referring to patients who had first developed the neurosis in childhood; both of the 'personality' descriptions might also apply to individuals suffering from long standing disorders of mood and obsessional symptomatology. Slater and Roth (1969) consider that there is a specificity about the obsessional personality structure which is characterized by its rigidity, inflexibility and lack of adaptability, its conscientiousness and love of order and discipline, and its persistence in the face of obstacles; it is, they state, characterized by a mental 'inertia', that is a difficulty in moving, but once set moving in a given direction, difficult to stop or deflect. They consider that this personality structure forms the basis of obsessional neurosis but they also note that many patients with involutional melancholia, anxiety states, and a variety of other neurotic disorders may also have shown such traits in their premorbid state. Beech and Liddell (1974) considered that one trait in particular might predispose to the development of the neurosis: a special alertness to the possibility of harmful consequences of interacting with the environment.

Black (1974) has undertaken a review of statements concerning the premorbid personality of patients suffering from obsessional neurosis; although methods of defining and assessing the traits varied from author to author, an absence of such traits was found in proportions varying from 16 per cent to 36 per cent of the samples surveyed. He pointed out that retrospective accounts of premorbid personality, by both the patients and their relatives, are liable to inaccuracy and distortion and he concluded his review with the opinion that the personality structure can only be one factor in determining the pattern of the subsequent neurosis.

Early precepts and examples received during childhood, like hereditary factors, are intimately bound up with concepts of the development of personality. It is sometimes held that obsessional neurotics have been subject to excessively strict training and high moral standards during childhood. Although such background influences might be expected, retrospective accounts by patients of their relationship with their parents are seldom reliable and are subject to unwitting falsification in an attempt by the patient to explain his present predicament. Using an advanced methodological design, the study by Siegelman (1974) showed this to be true for homosexual women and there is no reason to suppose the operation of such factors as a 'search after meaning' and apportionment of blame for the predicament would be any less in evidence for obsessional neurotics; so far the results of reliable prospective studies have not been reported.

The association of obsessions and organic brain disease

Obsessional symptomatology is sometimes reported in association with organic disease of the brain but, except in the case of post-encephalitic parkinsonism, this is probably no more than a chance occurrence. In a survey of patients suffering from obsessional neurosis, Grimshaw (1964) found that about one third of the patients had suffered in the past from various afflictions of the central nervous system; however, the majority of these were probably merely coincidental although, when compared with a control group, the incidence of Sydenham's chorea, meningitis, and encephalitis was higher. Pollitt (1969) surveyed the literature and concluded that the obsessional manifestations associated with organic brain disease are usually motor phenomena of a fairly primitive kind, such as the oculogyric crisis, and the movement itself preceded the subjective sense of compulsion to carry it out.

TREATMENT OF OBSESSIONAL NEUROSIS

Course and prognosis

The construction of a plan of treatment for any disorder must rest upon a knowledge of the natural history and prognosis of the untreated condition. The advent of a number of more effective treatments than were available in the past makes it necessary to rely on accounts of the natural history before such treatments were introduced.

Information regarding the course and outcome of obsessional neurosis have been summarized by Goodwin, Guze, and Robins (1969) and by Black (1974). In the first of these studies the findings of 13 published follow-up surveys were combined; two of the studies had been carried out in the United States, five in Britain, three in Scandinavian countries, and one each in Germany, Hong Kong, and Switzerland. Altogether these combined studies comprised the observations on more than 800 patients many of whom had been followed up for more than 15 years. The distillation of the findings were: that the onset was commonly around 20 years of age, that 65 per cent of all patients developed the illness before the age of 25, and that fewer than 15 per cent did so after the age of 35. Many authors have noted that the neurosis could develop as early as 6 years and Black produced a frequency polygraph of the ages of onset based upon eight published studies and concluded that the age of onset was before the age of 15 in one-third of the patients; however, this conclusion may have been influenced by the inclusion of two studies (those of Kringlen and of Skoog) in which patients suffering from obsessional neurosis and from phobic neurosis were combined, for it is possible that when these disorders are considered separately there would be a significant difference in the age of onset of the two neuroses. Black also concluded that significant life events are associated with the onset of obsessional neurosis in about half of the patients and, although there is considerable discrepancy in the findings of the various studies, sexual and marital difficulties, pregnancy, illness, or the death of a relative appear to be common precipitants.

The course of obsessional neurosis has been categorized by Ingram (1961) as being constant (static or worsening), fluctuating, or phasic. In the fluctuating type, periods of worsening are interspersed with relative improvement whereas in the phasic course there have been one or more periods of complete freedom from symptoms since the onset of the disorder. The latter group seems to resemble the 'endogenous obsessional neurosis' of Slater and Roth (1969) and is probably based upon an underlying cyclical affective disorder. Black tabulated the findings of three published studies; there was a relative agreement between these authors that a phasic course was observed in about 12 per cent of patients and a fluctuating course in about 30 per cent; the remainder, i.e. over 50 per cent of all the patients, showed a constant course.

Obsessional neurosis has long been considered to be more resistant to treatment and to have a poorer outcome than other neurotic syndromes; however, many authors have warned against taking too pessimistic a view which may be based upon biassed samples in psychiatric clinics. In their survey, Goodwin and his colleagues concluded that the prognosis is relatively favourable for patients with milder degrees of the disorder, 60 to 80 per cent being improved or free of symptoms one to five years after the diagnosis was first made. For more severe degrees of the neurosis, as judged by the need for hospital admission, the prognosis is less favourable and all that may be expected is a degree of improvement which occurs in about a third of the patients. Black could identify few prognostic indicators about which there was a general agreement between authors. Whereas some have identified certain features, such as mode of onset, premorbid personality, symptom pattern, and an admixture of other symptoms, as having a particular prognostic import, these conclusions have been contradicted by others. The only conclusion that can at present be drawn with any degree of confidence is the somewhat banal one that the longer the duration of the disorder the less good the prospect of ultimate recovery.

All these studies are based upon patients who received supportive treatment but little else in the way of specific therapy.

Assessment prior to treatment

The establishment of a therapeutic programme for a patient suffering from an obsessional neurosis must be preceded by a careful consideration of a number of important factors; if this procedure is skimped then mistakes may be made, the wrong approach will be adopted, and the best chances of recovery will be forgone. Of major importance in the assessment are the duration of symptoms and the attitudes of the patient and his relatives towards his disorder, the presence of other psychopathology, and the particular pattern of the obsessional symptomatology.

(a) A careful history is required of the course of the neurosis, at what age and in what circumstances symptoms first appeared and whether there have been periods of remission or amelioration of the condition; if improvement has occurred in the past an enquiry of possible factors related to this should be made.

(b) The attitude of the patient towards his disorder must be established; a special characteristic of the obsessional patient is his embarrassment about his own incomprehensibly foolish behaviour and this is certainly a factor which leads to the delay, perhaps of years, before he seeks help (Pollitt, 1960). His embarrassment may still lead him to minimize or rationalize his disorder even after he has come, or been brought, for treatment. This factor leads some patients to reject a therapeutic procedure which requires that they perform their ritualistic behaviour in front of others.

(c) The attitude of the spouse or parent to the patient's obsessional behaviour, the degree to which they collude with and maintain the behaviour and the quality of the relationship in general.

(d) The presence of other significant psychopathology, especially disorder of mood and whether the mood disorder is largely a reaction to the distress of the obsessional symptoms or whether it may be considered to be the prime generative source of the symptoms. If a mood disorder is present, an assessment of the relative degree of the components of depression, anxiety, and irritability must be undertaken and, as an aid to this, the completion of the Irritability-Depression-Anxiety (IDA) Scale (Snaith *et al.*, 1978) may be helpful.

(e) The pattern and triggering factors of all aspects of the obsessional symptoms should be ascertained. A superficial examination may only elicit the most prominent or distressing obsessional symptom and overlook the fact that other obsessional phenomena also occur. It is also essential to ascertain the circumstances which facilitate the symptom, e.g. does an obsessional ritual of checking the security of door locks only occur if the patient is in the house alone or does it occur whether or not the husband is also present? The completion of the Leyton Obsessional Inventory (Cooper, 1970) is helpful; from this are derived trait, symptom, resistance, and interference scores and a particularly helpful modification of the use of this instrument has been introduced by Robertson and Mulhall (1979) who have constructed a grid method of assessing the resistance and interference scores so that changes in these may be better evaluated according to circumstances (e.g. completed 'as I am at home' and 'as I am in hospital') and in response to any therapeutic procedure. It must be kept in mind that the patient's particular obsessional symptom may not appear in the Leyton Inventory and the value of the instrument would be further increased, especially when using the Robertson and Mulhall modification, by allowing space for the insertion of any other symptoms peculiar to the patient.

Therapeutic procedures

Behaviour therapy
A variety of techniques are now comprised under the rubric of behaviour therapy.

Wolpe (1958) considered that, for both his 'anxiety elevating' and 'anxiety reducing' obsessions, the technique of systematic densitization, during which anxiety is allayed whilst the patient is encouraged to think about or be in contact with increasing degrees of his feared circumstance, provided the 'crux of therapy'. However, this technique was not subjected to critical investigation and experiment and only rather sporadic reports appeared; Beech and Vaughan (1978) summarized the results of these reports: 21 patients were treated and considerable improvement occurred in just over a half of them. It appears that behaviour therapists were not encouraged by their experience with systematic desensitization and soon reports of a number of other techniques appeared.

Meyer (1966) put forward the view that the patient's expectation of a disastrous outcome, if he did not engage in his obsessional behaviour, could be modified if he was kept in contact with his feared circumstances and prevented from carrying out his accustomed ritual. He put this idea to the test on two patients, one of whom suffered from obsessional washing and the other from intrusive thoughts of a sexual and blasphemous nature; both patients had undergone previous attempts at treatment including systematic desensitization for the first and a leucotomy operation for the second. Both were treated in hospital. The nursing staff was instructed to prevent the obsessional washer from carrying out her rituals and during the therapeutic sessions she was brought deliberately into contact with the sources of her feared contamination. The second patient was instructed deliberately to engage in her thoughts of having intercourse with the 'Holy Ghost' for long periods of time. The first patient spent over three months in hospital and received over 20 hours of treatment in the therapeutic sessions whilst the second patient spent nine weeks in hospital and received 25 hours of treatment. At follow-up, which was at fourteen months and two years respectively, both the patients and their husbands considered that there had been some improvement but the account of the residual symptomatology suggests that this was of a very partial degree. A less sanguine therapist might have been discouraged but Dr Meyer considered a further trial of the method was warranted. Accordingly, together with colleagues (Meyer, Levy, and Schnurer, 1974) he developed the method and reported on the results of treatment of 11 patients suffering from obsessional neurosis with observable rituals. The treatment depended upon in-patient care and daily sessions with the therapist; nurses were instructed to carry out continual supervision during the waking hours and to prevent ritualistic behaviour by 'engaging the patient in other activities, discussion and very occasionally – and only with the patient's consent – mild physical restraint'. Staff, as well as patients, were given 'social reinforcement' for any improvement, in the form of praise by the therapist; two patients received small monetary rewards and encouragement and optimism were enhanced by meetings with patients who had been successfully treated. The therapist frequently demonstrated 'appropriate behaviour' and encouraged the patient to imitate him. After some symptomatic improvement the patient went home for increasing periods of time, sometimes in the company of a therapist or nurse and, when possible, relatives were instructed in methods of increasing the patient's control over unwanted behaviour. Follow-up assessments were carried out at periods varying from six months to six years after treatment; two patients were free of symptoms, six were much improved and two had shown no response to treatment. To this programme the name apotrepic therapy was given (Greek: *apotrepos*, turn away, dissuade, deter).

Various terms have been introduced for the techniques included in behaviour therapy of obsessions. The restraint imposed upon the patient from carrying out his obsessional behaviour is now usually called 'response prevention'. Encouraging the patient to observe the therapist engaging in contact with the feared circumstance is called 'modelling'; this may be 'passive modelling' when the patient merely observes, but is 'participant modelling' if he is persuaded to imitate the therapist (Röper, Rachman, and Marks, 1975). 'Shaping' is the term applied to the process of encouragement given to the patient for progressive approximation to the feared situation and 'flooding' refers to exposure to the feared situation at high intensity early in treatment. The instruction to the patient deliberately to engage in his obsessive thoughts for prolonged periods has been called 'satiation' (Rachman, 1976) and the term 'thought stopping' (attributed to Taylor by Wolpe, 1958) is the procedure by which the therapist interrupts a train of obsessional thinking by making a sharp sound or shouting some such word as 'stop'. A useful summary of these and other behavioural techniques has been made by Stern (1978a).

A series of studies on obsessional patients with observable rituals was carried out at The Maudsley Hospital, and the results of these studies have been summarized by Marks, Hodgson, and Rachman (1975). Twenty patients with a mean age of 35 and a mean duration of rituals of 10 years were treated as in-patients over periods of four to twelve weeks and received a mean of 23 treatment sessions each. Variations of the treatment techniques were used and patients were either gradually or quickly exposed to their feared circumstance at high intensity; for some patients a modelling procedure was incorporated into the treatment programme. There was no continuous observation by staff and response prevention was 'self-imposed' — that is, the patient was instructed not to carry out his ritual after the exposure session. The authors considered that reassurance given by others to the patient's anxious requests merely prolonged and reinforced the symptoms so that every request for reassurance was countered by some such statement as 'I cannot answer that'. At a two-year follow-up 14 patients were much improved and 5 were unchanged; most of the improvement in successful cases took place during the first three weeks of treatment. They concluded that the role of actual response prevention in the treatment programme is unknown, for their results were comparable with those of Meyer and his colleagues where response prevention was the keystone of therapy. The authors found no major differences in outcome according to whether the patient had been exposed slowly or rapidly to his feared circumstances or whether or not modelling was part of the treatment programme, but they stated that it is now their practice to expose the patient rapidly to his feared situation. They commented that a good working relationship between therapist and patient is essential and that no attempt should be made to push the patient at a faster pace than he consented to go. They also considered that co-operation and involvement of relatives in the programme is often crucial for success and that treatment may need to be continued in the patient's home after his discharge from hospital. They found that depression was usually associated with some increase in obsessional symptoms but that after treatment depression might occur without recurrence of the obsessions. Some patients were treated with tricyclic antidepressant drugs during or after the trial of behavioural treatments which may have introduced a confounding effect since the role of these drugs in treatment of obsessional neurosis is not fully evaluated.

The treatment of patients without observable rituals is generally held to be a more difficult proposition. Emmelkamp and Kwee (1977) subjected five patients to two procedures: 'thought stopping' and 'prolonged exposure in imagination'. They found some decrease in symptomatology after both programmes but no difference in effectiveness between them. Stern (1978b) subjected four patients to a thought-stopping programme; the patient was asked to ruminate on his obsessional theme as strongly as possible and after 30 seconds the therapist rapped the desk and at this signal the patient was instructed to shout 'Stop'. If tapping the desk did not disrupt the thought then the patient was instructed to twang an elastic band on his wrist, to switch his thoughts to a pleasant image and finally to achieve control by subvocal self-command. A further seven patients were subjected to a therapeutic programme termed 'satiation' which the author likens to the therapeutic technique of paradoxical intention. The patients were encouraged to ruminate on their obsessive thought as intensively as possible for an hour at a time, at first speaking the rumination out loud in the presence of the therapist. Two out of the seven patients who received the latter treatment showed worthwhile improvement but none of the four patients on the thought-stopping regime improved.

An uncommon variant of the obsessional paradigm has been designated by Rachman (1974) as primary obsessional slowness. He observed ten patients who were all extremely meticulous in carrying out their daily tasks. They all agreed that their behaviour was unacceptable and that it consumed an inordinate amount of time. The author instituted a therapeutic programme which combined 'prompting' and 'external pacing', by which the patient was encouraged by the therapist to carry out activities more quickly, combined with the technique of shaping in which the therapist strongly encouraged improvements in the time taken to carry out tasks. He found that, by the use of this programme, there were strong, early improvements followed by a long period of slow, steady gains interspersed with periods during which improvement did not occur.

A major drawback of the therapeutic techniques described above is the considerable amount of therapists' time involved and the training and co-operation of the many members of hospital staff who may be in contact with the patient. Such facilities may only be present in certain centres where there is a high degree of interest and enthusiasm for the treatment. Moreover, some of the techniques may only be appropriate if the obsessional symptoms are manifest when the patient is in contact with the therapist but if this is not the case, the use of the therapeutic techniques described above may not be possible. As an instance of this sort of problem a man, who was involved as a driver of long-distance heavy road transport, lost an hour or more a day and stood in threat of dismissal from his job. About once a day when he had driven past a cyclist the thought occurred to him that he may have harmed or killed him. He was unable to stop his vehicle until the next lay-by which might be several miles further on but when he had found such a stopping place he had to dismount and walk back along the road until he saw the cyclist, unharmed, approaching him. In hospital no such obsessional thought occurred to him and the proposition that a therapist should accompany him on his daily work was a practical impossibility. For such a situation, and possibly also for the generality of obsessional symptoms, there remain the techniques of carrying out the therapeutic programme entirely in imagination. Such techniques are the 'covert sensitization' of Cautela (1967) and its variant, 'covert reinforcement' (Cautela, 1970). The term 'covert' in this context implies that the patient imagines himself to be involved in the circumstances which call forth his obsession. In the technique of covert sensitization the patient is instructed to imagine the circumstances of his obsessional behaviour and when he signals that he has obtained a clear image the therapist suggests to him that he is experiencing some unpleasant sensation such as nausea. In the alternative procedure of covert reinforcement the patient's signal of a clear image is followed by the suggestion that he is leaving his obsessional circumstances and experiencing some pleasant sensation. So far there have been only isolated reports of the treatment of obsessional neurosis by such techniques (Lambley, 1974; Wisocki, 1970) but if the effectiveness of the method were to be established there is the possibility of treating patients for whom the establishment of other behavioural therapeutic programmes would pose insurmountable problems.

Drug treatment

Sedative drugs have only a small role in the treatment of obsessional neurosis. Taken continuously they rapidly produce habituation and lose their effect but sometimes a patient may be helped by a sedative taken shortly before he encounters his feared circumstance; such drugs will therefore only help those patients who experience their obsessional symptoms in specific circumstances at occasional intervals; all sedatives such as the barbiturates and benzodiazepine tranquillizers may increase irritability (Ingram and Timbury, 1960) and since Beech has pointed out that the mood change of irritability often triggers the obsessional symptoms, the patient's condition may be worsened rather than improved by the prevalent habit of prescription of continuous medication with such drugs. Phenothiazine drugs with sedative effects, such as chlorpromazine, may be indicated when obsessions occur in the setting of severe depressive agitation although usually the treatment of the depression itself with an antidepressant drug will be the better procedure.

Most writers on the treatment of obsessional neurosis (*inter alia* Marks, 1973; Beech and Vaughan, 1978) consider that there is a role for the use of antidepressant drugs in obsessional neurosis and this is certainly the first step to be undertaken when any degree of primary depressive illness underlies the obsessional symptoms. Although there is at present a vogue to treat obsessional neurosis with clomipramine, sometimes by intravenous infusion, there have been no careful clinical trials to establish the superiority of this particular drug or route of administration and there are no present grounds for the belief that the chlorine atom tacked on to the imipramine nucleus produces a specific 'anti-obsessional' effect lacking in other tricyclic antidepressants. Among the few controlled clinical trials that have been undertaken in this field is that of Rachman and his colleagues (1979). These workers used a 2×2 factorial design of behaviour therapy *versus* relaxation and clomipramine *versus* a placebo drug; they concluded that clomipramine treatment was followed by several broad improvements and that it appeared that the mood-regulating effect of the drug was the cause of the secondary improvement in obsessional rituals. They noted that significant depression probably maintained obsessional symptoms but a correction of the mood disorder was not always followed by a decline in the obsessional symptoms. It should be noted that Rachman and his colleagues prescribed the tricyclic drug in a dose increasing to 225 mg daily and it may be that the poor results that many clinicians have experienced with antidepressant drug therapy may partly be due to a reluctance to prescribe the drug in adequate dosage.

Physical treatments

Electroconvulsive therapy can only be expected to improve obsessional symptoms when they occur in the setting of depressive illness and Sargant and Slater (1971) have pointed out that, when this is not the case, obsessional symptoms may be made worse by ECT. However, this should not deter the therapist from using the treatment when depression, which has not responded to drug therapy, is clearly a feature of the clinical picture.

Improvements have recently taken place in the surgical treatment of mental illness and with present-day techniques it is possible to relieve mental disorder with little or no impairment of healthy mental function or other major unwanted effects. Indeed, after successful surgical treatment the whole quality of psychic life will improve since it is no longer dominated by the distressing morbid symptoms.

The results of surgical treatment for obsessional neurosis up until 1960 have been summarized by Sternberg (1974). Combined results from seven studies showed a good outcome in about half the patients. Such results, however, were not good enough to sustain interest in this approach to treatment and enthusiasm for psychosurgery waned. However, surgical treatment has continued in some centres and is practised quite widely in Britain (*British Medical Journal*, 1978). By 1951 Knight had introduced the modified operation based upon the orbital undercutting approach of Scoville. The study of the outcome of this procedure, which in one centre was used in 350 patients over a period of ten years, was a decided step towards a more critical assessment of surgical procedures (Sykes and Tredgold, 1964); the sample contained only 24 patients suffering from obsessional neurosis and on the whole these patients did not do so well as those suffering from depressive and anxiety states. A retrospective study was undertaken by Tan, Marks, and Marset (1971) in which 24 patients who had undergone psychosurgery were compared with matched patients who had not; the follow-up period was five years. Twenty-three of the patients had undergone a bimedial leucotomy and one patient had an orbital undercutting operation. It was reported that the surgical patients had a better outcome than the controls with respect to both obsessions and anxiety. Obsessions were reduced from a severe to a moderate degree of handicap, work adjustment improved and personality changes after operation were mild and not related to outcome.

More recently, stereotactic techniques have been introduced in order to locate the lesion more precisely and to minimize unwanted effects. Ström-Olsen and Carlisle (1971) reported upon Knight's technique of implanting radioactive yttrium seeds in the posterior orbital cortex, their sample contained 20 patients suffering from obsessional neurosis of whom 10 showed complete recovery or marked improvement and a further three showed some improvement. A further review of this technique appeared some years later (Göktepe, Young, and Bridges, 1975) and again, over a minimum follow-up period of two years, 7 out of 18 obsessional patients showed complete recovery and 8 lesser degrees of recovery; only 3 were unchanged and none were worse. Fifteen of these 18 patients had been ill for more than four years before operation and it was found that outcome was not related to the duration of illness.

There had been earlier suggestions that lesions placed in the anterior cingulum were more beneficial in the case of obsessional neurosis (Lewin, 1961). The development of a stereotactic technique at the Atkinson Morley's hospital in London included placement of lesions both in the cingulum and the lower medial quadrants of the frontal lobes. This technique was called stereotactic limbic leucotomy and Mitchell-Heggs, Kelly, and Richardson (1976) reported upon the outcome with this approach. The follow-up period was relatively short (16 months) but 7 out of 27 patients suffering from obsessional neurosis were symptom free whilst 11 were reported to be much improved and 2 to be improved. Such results are marginally better than those reported with the stereotactic tractotomy technique but against this must be set the record that two patients were reported to be worse after the limbic leucotomy. In general, adverse effects of the operation were very low and unwelcome effects on the personality were not noted by either the patients or their relatives.

At the present time it may be said that although the psychotherapeutic approaches to the treatment of obsessional neurosis allow for more optimism than was previously the case and although pharmacotherapy has also contributed to the improved outlook, none the less a considerable amount of chronicity still results from the condition. This being the case the patient who has suffered from severely handicapping obsessional neurosis continuously for five years or longer and who has not responded to other therapeutic approaches should be carefully reassessed and then offered the chance of improvement with psychosurgery; cure can of course not be guaranteed but the patient may be informed that the likelihood of a worsening of his condition is remote whereas the chance of marked symptom relief is high and he may also be informed that with modern surgical techniques deleterious effects upon his personality do not now occur.

References

*AKHTAR, S., WIG, N. N., VARMA, V. K., PERSHOD, D., and VERMA, S. K. (1975). A phenomenological analysis of symptoms of obsessive-compulsive neurosis. *Br. J. Psychiat*. **127**, 342–9.

BARRACLOUGH, B. M. and MITCHELL-HEGGS, N. A. (1978). Use of neurosurgery for psychological disorder in British Isles during 1974–6. *Br. med. J*. **ii**, 1591–4.

BEECH, H. R. (1971). Ritualistic activity in obsessional patients. *J. Psychosom. Res*. **15**, 417–22.

*—— (1974). Approaches to understanding obsessional states. In *Obsessional states* (ed. H. R. Beech). Methuen, London.

—— and LIDDELL, A. (1974). Decision-making, mood states and ritualistic behaviour among obsessional patients. In *Obsessional states* (ed. H. R. Beech). Methuen, London.

—— and PERIGAULT, J. (1974). Toward a theory of obsessional disorder. In *Obsessional states* (ed. H. R. Beech). Methuen, London.

—•— and VAUGHAN, M. (1978). *Behavioural treatment of obsessional states*. Wiley, London.

*BLACK, A. (1974). The natural history of obsessional neurosis. In *Obsessional states* (ed. H. R. Beech). Methuen, London.

BROWN, F. W. (1942). Hereditary in the psychoneuroses. *Proc. R. Soc. Med*. **35**, 785–90.

CAUTELA, J. R. (1967). Covert sensitization. *Psychol. Rep*. **20**, 459–68.

—— (1970). Covert reinforcement. *Behav. Ther*. **1**, 33–50.

COOPER, J. (1970). The Leyton Obsessional Inventory. *Psychol. Med*. **1**, 48–65.

EMMELKAMP, P. M. G. and KWEE, K. G. (1977). Obsessional ruminations: a comparison between thought-stopping and prolonged exposure in imagination. *Behav. Res. Ther*. **15**, 441–4.

EYSENCK, H. J. and RACHMAN, S. (1965). *The causes and cures of neurosis*. Routledge and Kegan Paul, London.

FREUD, S. (1896). Further remarks on the neuropsychoses of defence. In *Standard edition of the complete psychological works*, Vol. 3 (ed. J. Strachey). The Hogarth Press, London.

—— (1908). Character and anal erotism. In *Standard edition of the complete psychological works*, Vol. 9 (ed. J. Strachey). The Hogarth Press, London.

—— (1926). Inhibitions, symptoms and anxiety. In *Standard edition of the complete psychological works*, Vol. 20 (ed. J. Strachey). The Hogarth Press, London.

FENICHEL, O. (1946). *The psychoanalytic theory of neurosis*. Kegan Paul, Trench and Trubner, London.

GITTLESON, N. L. (1966a). The effects of obsessions on depressive psychosis. *Br. J. Psychiat.* 112, 253–8.

—— (1966b). The phenomenology of obsessions in depressive psychosis. *Br. J. Psychiat.* 112, 261–4.

—— (1966c). The fate of obsessions in depressive psychosis. *Br. J. Psychiat.* 112, 705–8.

GÖKTEPE, E. O., YOUNG, L. B., and BRIDGES, P. K. (1975). A further review of the results of stereotactic subcaudate tractotomy. *Br. J. Psychiat.* 126, 270–81.

GOODWIN, D. W., GUZE, S. B., and ROBINS, E. (1969). Follow-up studies in obsessional neurosis. *Archs gen. Psychiat.* 220, 182–7.

GRIMSHAW, L. (1964). Obsessional disorder and neurological illness. *J. Neurosurg. Psychiat.* 27, 229–31.

INGRAM, I. M. (1969). Obsessional illness in mental hospital patients. *J. ment. Sci.* 107, 1035–42.

—— and TIMBURY, G. C. (1960). The side-effects of Librium. *Lancet* ii, 766.

KRÄUPL TAYLOR, F. (1966). *Psychopathology, its causes and symptoms*. Butterworth, London.

LAMBLEY, P. (1974). Differential effects of psychotherapy and behavioural techniques in acute obsessive-compulsive disorder. *Br. J. Psychiat.* 125, 181–3.

LEIGH, D., PARE, C. M. B., and MARKS, J. (1977). *A concise encyclopaedia of psychiatry*. MTP Press, Lancaster.

LEWIN, W. (1961). Observations on selected leucotomy. *J. Neurol. Neurosurg. Psychiat.* 24, 37–44.

LEWIS, A. J. (1934). Melancholia: a clinical survey of depressive states. *J. ment. Sci.* 80, 277–378. [Reprinted in *Inquiries in psychiatry*. Routledge and Kegan Paul, London (1967).]

—— (1936). Problems of obsessional illness. *Proc. R. Soc. Med.* 29, 325–36. [Reprinted in *Inquiries in psychiatry*. Routledge and Kegan Paul, London (1967).]

—— (1957). Obsessional illness. *Acta neuropsiq. argent.* 3, 323–35. [Reprinted in *Inquiries in psychiatry*. Routledge and Kegan Paul, London (1967).]

MAKHLOUF-NORRIS, and NORRIS, H. (1972). The obsessive compulsive syndrome as a neurotic device. *Br. J. Psychiat.* 121, 277–88.

MARKS, I. M. (1969). *Fears and phobias*. Heinemann, London.

—— (1973). New approaches to the treatment of obsessive–compulsive disorders. *J. nerv. ment. Dis.* **156**, 420–62.

*—— HODGSON, R. J. and RACHMAN, S. (1975). Treatment of chronic obsessive–compulsive neurosis by *in vivo* exposure: a two year follow-up and issues in treatment. *Br. J. Psychiat.* **127**, 349–64.

*MEYER, V. (1966). Modification of expectations in cases with obsessional rituals. *Behav. Res. Ther.* **4**, 273–80.

—— and CHESSER, E. S. (1970). *Behaviour therapy in clinical psychiatry.* Penguin, Harmondsworth.

*—— LEVY, R., and SCHNURER, A. (1974). The behavioural treatment of obsessive–compulsive disorders. In *Obsessional states* (ed. H. R. Beech). Methuen, London.

MILLAR, D. G. (1980). A repertory grid study of obsessionality: distinctive cognitive structure or distinctive cognitive element? *Br. J. Med. Psychol.* **53**, 59–66.

MITCHELL-HEGGS, N., KELLY, D., and RICHARDSON, A. (1976). Stereotactic limbic leucotomy—a follow-up after 16 months. *Br. J. Psychiat.* **128**, 226–41.

*MORAN, E. (1970). Varieties of pathological gambling. *Br. J. Psychiat.* **116**, 593–7.

POLLITT, J. (1960). Natural history studies in mental illness: a discussion based upon a pilot study of obsessional states. *J. ment. Sci.* **106**, 93–113.

—— (1969). Obsessional states. *Br. J. hosp. Med.* **2**, 1146–50.

RACHMAN, S. (1974). Primary obsessional slowness. *Behav. Res. Ther.* **12**, 9–18.

—— (1976). The modification of obsessions, a new formulation. *Behav. Res. Ther.* **14**, 437–43.

—— COBB, J., GREY, S., McDONALD, B., MAWSON, D., SARTORY, G., and STERN, R. (1979). Behavioural treatment of obsessive-compulsive disorders with and without clomipramine. *Behav. Res. Ther.* **17**, 467–78.

RICKLES, N. K. (1942). Exhibitionism. *J. nerv. ment. Dis.* **95**, 11–17.

ROBERTSON, J. R. and MULHALL, D. J. (1979). The clinical evaluation of obsessionality: a development of the Leyton Obsessional Inventory. *Psychol. Med.* **9**, 147–55.

*ROOTH, F. G. (1971). Indecent exposure and exhibitionism. *Br. J. hosp. Med.* **5**, 521–33.

RÖPER, G., RACHMAN, S., and MARKS, I. M. (1975). Passive and participant modelling in exposure treatment of obsessive compulsive neurotics. *Behav. Res. Ther.* **13**, 271–9.

RÜDIN, E. (1953). Ein Beitrag zur Frage Zwangskrankheit insbesondere ihre hereditären Beziehungen. *Arch. Psychiat. NervKrankh.* **191**, 14–54.

SARGANT, W. and SLATER, E. (1977). *Introduction to physical methods of treatment in psychiatry.* 8th edn. Churchill Livingstone, Edinburgh.

SCHNEIDER, K. (1925). Zwangszustände und Schizophrenie. *Arch. Psychiat. NervKrankh.* **74**, 93–107.

SIEGELMAN, M. (1974). Parental background of homosexual and heterosexual women. *Br. J. Psychiat.* **124**, 14–21.

SLATER, E. and ROTH, M. (1969). *Clinical psychiatry*, 3rd edn. Baillière, Tindall and Cassell, London.

SNAITH, R. P., CONSTANTOPOULOS, A. A., JARDINE, M. Y., and McGUFFIN, P. (1978). A clinical scale for the self-assessment of irritability. *Br. J. Psychiat.* **132**, 164–72.

STENGEL, E. (1945). A study on the clinical aspects of the relationship between obsessional neurosis and psychotic reaction types. *J. ment. Sci.* **91**, 166–87.

STERN, R. S. (1978a). *Behavioural techniques*. Academic Press, London.

—— (1978b). Obsessive thoughts: the problem of therapy. *Br. J. Psychiat.* **133**, 200–6.

*—— and COBB, J. P. (1978). Phenomenology of obsessive–compulsive neurosis. *Br. J. Psychiat.* **132**, 233–40.

STERNBERG, M. (1974). Physical treatment in obsessional disorders. In *Obsessional states* (ed. H. R. Beech). Methuen, London.

STROM-OLSEN, R. and CARLISLE, S. (1971). Bifrontal stereotactic tractotomy: a follow-up study of its effects on 210 patients. *Br. J. Psychiat.* **118**, 141–54.

SYKES, M. K. and TREDGOLD, R. F. (1964). Restricted orbital undercutting. *Br. J. Psychiat.* **110**, 609–40.

TAN, E., MARKS, I. M., and MARSET, P. (1971). Bimedial leuctomy in obsessive-compulsive neurosis: a controlled serial enquiry. *Br. J. Psychiat.* **118**, 155–64.

TEASDALE, J. D. (1974). Learning models of obsessional–compulsive disorder. In *Obsessional states* (ed. H. R. Beech). Methuen, London.

VEITH, I. (1965). *Hysteria: the history of a disease*. Phoenix Books; University of Chicago Press, Illinois.

*WALKER, V. J. (1973). Explanation in obsessional neurosis. *Br. J. Psychiat.* **123**, 675–80.

—— and BEECH, H. R. (1969). Mood state and ritualistic behaviour of obsessional patients. *Br. J. Psychiat.* **115**, 1261–8.

WISOCKI, P. A. (1970). Treatment of obsessive–compulsive behaviour by covert sensitization and covert reinforcement. *J. Behav. Ther. exp. Psychiat.* **1**, 233–9.

WOLPE, J. (1958). *Psychotherapy by reciprocal inhibition*. Stanford University Press, California.

4

Hysteria and hypochondriasis

HYSTERIA and hypochondriasis are concepts of disease which both have their origins in antiquity; throughout the ages views about their nature and attributes have changed and fluctuated and may be seen to reflect the historical evolution of attitudes towards the psychic manifestations of disease, the interface between body and soul, in the medical corpus. The phenomena of both disorders are based on normal mental processes, present in the healthy as well as the sick; the one a tendency to dissociate and the other a fear of sickness and death. Their elaboration into disease entities may be seen as an attempt by doctors to structuralize and name and thereby deal with uncomfortable psychological attributes which all men recognize within themselves. At times hysteria and hypochondriasis have been regarded as respected diseases, at other times as manifestations of evil powers and yet again as foolish behaviour of no account. They have been regarded as separate disorders and then again as the same disorder manifested in the separate sexes, so that in the seventeenth century Thomas Sydenham wrote:

> However much antiquity may have laid the blame of hysteria upon the uterus, hypochondriasis (which we impute to some obstruction of the spleen or viscera) is as like it, as one egg is to another.

HYSTERIA

Hysteria yesterday

The concept of hysteria has undergone many transmutations and is still used in a great variety of senses. The term is directly derived from the Greek *hystera*, the uterus, but beliefs that the origin of certain symptoms were caused by migration of that organ to unaccustomed parts of the body antedated Greek medicine by many centuries. Such a belief may have originated from the fact that in certain disorders of the limbic lobe of the brain, such as temporal lobe epilepsy, the fit may be preceded by a mood disorder characterized by anxiety accompanied by a sensation of a swelling rising upward through the body. This last symptom has been enshrined under the venerable term 'globus hystericus' and its association with turbulent emotion and sexuality is expressed in Shakespeare's *King Lear*:

> O, how this mother swells up toward my heart!
> *Hysterica passio*, down, thou climbing sorrow
> Thy element's below.

The history of changing concepts about hysteria is interwoven with femininity (and the attitudes to that sex of male physicians), fecundity, erotic disorganization, turbulent emotion, and dramatic symptoms; this history has been brilliantly written by Ilza Veith (1965) and the author is indebted to that work for most of the historical material up until the time of Freud.

With the increasing domination of European thought by ecclesiastical teaching, the supposed evil of erotic pleasure was expounded to the detriment of the view of sexual expression as a natural function. So closely had been the presumed association between sexuality and the disorders called 'hysterical' that the belief arose that those who manifested such symptoms were in league with the forces of evil, if not possessed by the Devil himself. It was inevitable that, in such a climate of thought, attitudes should undergo a stark change from the view of the sufferer beset by emotional troubles and deserving of medical help to that of a miscreant, more or less wilfully wicked, whose fate should be punishment if not death; the vocation of the official known as the 'common pricker' was to 'diagnose' witchcraft by detecting areas of anaesthesia upon the skin of the unfortunate woman. In the late Middle Ages these views were challenged and among the daring voices was that of Phillipus Theophrastus Bombastus von Hohenheim, known as Paracelsus, who listed hysteria among the mental disorders that deprive man of his reason and wrote:

> The present-day clergy of Europe attribute such diseases to ghostly beings and three-fold spirits; we are not inclined to believe them.

An English physician, Edward Jordan (1578–1632) joined in the refutation of the demonological origin of symptoms; furthermore he argued that the source of symptoms arose in the brain and not in the uterus, thus presaging the neurological phase in the history of ideas surrounding hysteria, and he advocated a therapeutic approach based upon the release of emotional tension which he believed was the cause of the disorder.

The great physician, Thomas Sydenham (1624–89), also firmly included hysteria among the afflictions of the mind and he underlined the concepts of simulation and protean manifestations when he wrote:

> Few of the diseases of miserable mortality are not imitated by it.

A firm view of hysteria as a disorder of polysymptomatic presentation was typified by the Scottish physician, Robert Whytt (1714–66); he included, among the frequent manifestations of hysteria paroxysms, sensations of cold, trembling, a feeling of oppression, fleeting pains, protracted headaches, fainting, catalepsy, wind in the stomach, nervous and spasmodic asthma, nervous cough, giddiness, dimness of vision, and low spirits. In the eighteenth and nineteenth centuries, hysteria was tending to become a fashionable disease and the American, Benjamin Rush (1745–1813), was to expostulate:

> The Hysteric and Hypochondriacal disorders, once peculiar to the chambers of the great, are now to be found in our kitchens and workshops. All these diseases have been produced by our having deserted the simple diet and manners of our ancestors.

Baron von Feuchtersleben (1806–49), who introduced the term psychosis, also considered that hysteria occurred primarily among the overprivileged and effete. His contemporary and compatriot, Wilhelm Griesinger underlined the adverse traits of personality which were thought to be inextricably mingled with the symptoms of the disorder; an inclination towards deception and prevarication, jealousy, malice, and other personal failings; he also wrote of another concept which has intermittently been linked with hysteria, that of the noisy expression of turbulent emotion so that the most advanced cases:

> Manifest themselves by vociferation, singing, cursing, aimless wandering . . . attempts at suicide, nymphomaniacal excitment . . . noisy, perverse but still coherent actions . . . they retain but slight remembrance of what took place during the disorder.

The concept of hysteria as a gain-motivated disorder was expressed

by many, including Weir Mitchell (1829–1914); during his experience in the American Civil War he wrote:

> Cases of nostalgia, homesickness, were serious additions to the perils of
> wounds and disease . . . an interesting psychic malady, making men
> hysteric and incurable except by discharge [from the army].

Here, of course, it is the disorder nostalgia which is discussed, but its
links with hysteria were made plain.

The French neurologist and physician, Jean-Martin Charcot,
became interested in hysteria towards the end of the nineteenth
century. He added little to knowledge about the disorder except that
he firmly announced that hysteria was not the prerogative of the
female sex:

> Keep it well in mind and this should not require a great effort, that the
> word 'hysteria' means nothing, and little by little you will acquire the
> habit of speaking of hysteria in man without thinking of the uterus.

His disciple Pierre Janet (1907) devoted much study to hysteria,
basing his writings on close and careful observation. He denied the
prevalent concept of the sexual origin of hysteria and concentrated
his attention upon the subconscious ideas, the *idées fixes*, which he
believed to underly the 'hysterical accidents' or symptomatic ex-
pressions of the disorder. He recognized the work of his 'Austrian
colleagues' (Breuer and Freud) but claimed priority in drawing
attention to the necessity of bringing to consciousness the provoca-
tive event underlying hysteria. Janet's great contribution to the study
of hysteria was his emphasis on the mental mechanism of dissociation, a term which he seems to have been the first to use. He wrote:

> Hysteria is a malady of personal synthesis . . . a form of mental de-
> pression characterized by retraction of the field of consciousness and a
> tendency to dissociation and emancipation of the systems of ideas and
> functions that constitute personality. . . . The starting point of hysteria
> is the same as that of most great neuroses, it is a depression, an exhaustion
> of the higher centres of the encephalon.

He cited as causes of such exhaustion, puberty, diseases, and
emotion itself.

Sigmund Freud came to the study of hysteria, and indeed of
psychiatry, when a colleague, Joseph Breuer, recounted to him the
case history of a patient, Anna O., whom he was treating by hypnosis.

This patient suffered from symptoms which were found to be related to significant traumata in her life, including the illness and death of her father. Their study which they published in *Studien über Hysterie*, returned to the ancient themes of sexuality and repressed emotion in the genesis of hysteria, but a further theme was developed: that of the symbolic nature of the symptoms. It has been pointed out (Veith, p. 263) that, like those before him, Freud had no definition of the concept of hysteria and that when he travelled to Nancy to study the hypnotic treatment of Bernheim and Liébault, there seems to have been a stereotyped idea of the hysteric in existence which required no further definition. This tendency for a stereotyped idea of hysteria to develop, which none the less changed in pattern from one generation to the next was recognized by Pierre Janet when he wrote:

> Charcot described a type of hysteric that disappeared with him; nobody nowadays describes attacks of hysteria like Charcot did. . . . No doubt our types of hysterical phenomena are ephemeral, like his.

Hysteria today

The foregoing brief historical survey has introduced the multiple concepts associated with the ill-defined manifestations of a supposed disease, hysteria. It is clear from the lunch table talk of psychiatrists that most of these concepts are alive and well today although the disorder has received a formal definition in the Glossary of the 9th Revision of the *International classification of diseases*:

> 300.1   Hysteria. Mental disorders in which motives, of which the patient seems unaware, produce either a restriction of the field of consciousness or disturbances of motor or sensory function which may seem to have psychological advantage or symbolic value. It may be characterized by conversion phenomena or dissociative phenomena. In the conversion form the chief or only symptoms consist of psychogenic disturbance of function in some part of the body, e.g. paralysis, tremor, blindness, deafness, seizures. In the dissociative variety, the most prominent feature is a narrowing of the field of consciousness which seems to serve an unconscious purpose and is commonly accompanied or followed by selective amnesia. There may be dramatic but essentially superficial changes of personality sometimes taking the form of a fugue (wandering state). Behaviour may mimic psychosis, or rather the patient's idea of a psychosis.

This definition, arrived at by a committee, does its best to grapple with the multiple concepts; it is of interest that the so-called hysterical personality is now excluded from the definition; also anorexia nervosa, which was earlier classified under hysteria. Even so, a number of possibly unrelated concepts are brought together in the definition. Chodoff and Lyons (1958) have summarized the concepts of hysteria currently used in the United States. They are:

1. A pattern of behaviour habitually exhibited by certain individuals who are said to be hysterical personalities.
2. A particular kind of psychosomatic symptomatology called conversion hysteria or conversion reactions.
3. A psychoneurotic disorder characterized by phobias and anxiety manifestations: anxiety hysteria.
4. A particular psychopathological pattern.
5. A term of opprobrium.

Of these uses, the third is derived from Freud's term for a neurotic disorder, now usually called phobic neurosis, and the fourth is used as a diagnostic label for an individual with a 'particular psycho-sexual history' which the authors do not further elucidate. The opprobrium or pejorative context of the use of the term is also linked to a sense of therapeutic exasperation best expressed in the words of Slater and Glithero (1965):

> It is certain that some clinicians make the diagnosis of hysteria more readily than others. In some sense it is true to say that 'hysteria' is a label assigned to a particular relationship between the observer and the observed; it appears on the case sheet most readily if the doctor has found himself at a loss, if the case is obscure or if the treatment has been unsuccessful. Of all diagnoses it is that which is least likely to have been made in a spirit of detachment.

The concepts associated with hysteria will now be considered separately.

Personality disorder

Chodoff and Lyons surveyed the literature and found that the following traits had, at various times, been associated with the concept of the hysterical personality:

1. Egoism, vanity, egocentricity, self-indulgence;
2. Exhibitionism, dramatization, lying;
3. Unbridled display of affects, excitability, inconstancy;
4. Emotional shallowness;
5. Lascivious sexualization of all non-sexual functions;
6. Sexual frigidity, sexual immaturity.

Surveying this list they commented that what emerges is 'a picture of women in the words of men, a caricature of femininity'. In their own study of 17 patients they found no definite relationship between hysterical symptoms and particular personality traits of a type which might be termed 'hysterical'. Ziegler, Imboden, and Meyer (1960) also arrived at the conclusion that the 'hysterical' personality pattern was not a prerequisite for the occurrence of conversion symptoms and that the conventional concept of the personality type comprised such a scattered constellation of traits that it was clearly not a consistent entity. They sought to limit consideration of an underlying personality structure to just one trait: the expression of a tendency to role-playing, the so-called histrionic personality (Greek: *histrio*, an actor). Whilst admitting that most people tend to enact roles, the histrionic person does so in an unconvincing manner, the enactment varying from one situation to another and causing evident difficulties in forming relationships and stable social identities.

Ljungberg (1957) also considered the relationship of personality structure to symptomatic presentation in a study of hysteria. He defined the hysterical personality in the same context as Janet had done, a type dominated by suggestibility and distractibility; he also considered other personality traits and patterns which bordered on the abnormal, e.g. the psycho-infantile type, characterized by increased dependency on others, and the psychasthenic type in which a reduced supply of psychic energy is the most characteristic feature. In his study of 381 propositi he found that 43 per cent of the men and 47 per cent of the women exhibited an abnormality of personality but that no one type predominated. Eysenck (1960) has attempted to establish that patients suffering from hysteria are more extraverted and less neurotic than patients in whom the clinical picture is dominated by anxiety and depression, but this conclusion is not surprising in view of the tendency of psychiatrists to attach the label of hysteria to people whose personality structure is flamboyant and demonstrative and who are therefore likely to have a score in the direction of extraversion on the Maudsley Personality Inventory. Ingham and Robinson (1964) repeated the study, using the Maudsley Inventory, on patients diagnosed as hysteric who had been divided into two groups: those with predominant symptoms and those with predominant disorder of personality. They found that the personality disordered were indeed more extraverted than dysthymics, in keeping with Eysenck's hypothesis, but this difference was not found between those with predominant hysterical symptoms and the dysthymic patients with predominant anxiety and depression.

Multiple symptomatology

The presentation of a disorder in terms of multiple symptoms is one of the historical themes of hysteria. Recently a major effort has been made by workers at St. Louis in the USA, to redefine hysteria in terms of multiple symptoms over a protracted course of time (Farley, Woodruff, and Guze, 1968; Perley and Guze, 1962; Woodruff, 1967). The disorder they defined they renamed Briquet's syndrome; Briquet was a French physician who, in 1859, described a disorder characterized by many symptoms in different organ systems which defied medical explanation and was presumed to be hysterical in nature. The syndrome defined by the St. Louis group is similarly based on three criteria: first the patient must demonstrate a dramatic or complicated medical history beginning before the age of 35; second she must admit to 25 symptoms in nine out of ten symptom areas; third there must be no other diagnosis to explain the symptoms. The authors of this syndrome found it to be common, occurring in 1–2 per cent of the female population and to have a strong familial bias, occurring in 20 per cent of first-degree relatives of index cases. Apparently the disorder does not occur in males or if it does, the authors, true to historical attitudes towards hysteria, have not paid the matter much attention. Whilst accepting that such a condition exists and possibly accounts for a certain proportion of patients who circulate around the out-patient halls of hospitals throughout the world, there are nevertheless grave difficulties in defining a syndrome in such a way (Snaith, 1968) and a leading article in *The Lancet* (1977) considered that the description of Briquet's syndrome, or more correctly the St. Louis syndrome, was no substitute for hysteria.

Suggestion and communicability

That 'hysterics' are suggestible is another key theme which emerges from the historical survey. Consequently any psychological disorder which occurs under the influence of suggestion is liable to be placed in the diagnostic category of hysteria. In this way phenomena such as *folie à deux* and symptoms occurring in patients which are very similar in site and nature to the symptoms of a sick or deceased relative are readily considered to be hysterical in nature, as also are symptoms which appear in the wake of publicity about some disease which has been discovered in the neighbourhood in which the patient lives. Bizarre behaviour occurring in large or small groups of people under the influence of strong emotion is also usually considered to be hysterical; such were the dancing manias ar.J processions of flagellants in the Middle Ages; a more modern equivalent of the same phenomenon is the screaming frenzy and fainting fits of groups of young people at the long-awaited appearance of some pop star idol.

The most interesting of these manifestations is the so-called epidemic hysteria (*British Medical Journal*, 1979). These outbreaks appear sporadically among gatherings of young people and have been reported in the recent decades from many areas of the world. Girls make up the great majority of those affected and symptoms may be both physical, such as abdominal pain, or take the form of disordered and uncontrolled emotional display. The epidemic may commence dramatically in the setting of general concern about the outbreak of some disease in the neighbourhood or it may be instigated by a girl of considerable influence in her peer group; an example of the latter situation has been described by Benaim, Horder, and Anderson (1973) and the authors were able to obtain the later 'confession' of the instigator.

Mayou (1975) carried out an interesting survey of the personal and social situations in which phenomena of a hysterical type appear and he pointed out that, at various times and in different cultures, the same phenomena may be either socially approved or regarded as deviant or as evidence of illness; he suggested that the main focus of enquiry should now be directed away from the psychological mechanism of symptom formation and directed towards the question of why certain people in certain situations react with such inappropriate behaviour.

Gain and communication

Central to the concept of hysteria today is the possibility that the patient is deriving some advantage from the disorder. It is usually considered that there are two types of gain resulting from neurosis, the primary and the secondary gain. Primary gain is the relief from emotional conflict that the appearance of the symptom brings about; for example, underlying an episode of amnesia there may be a personal situation fraught with anxiety and the 'forgetting' of the situation relieves the distress but the amnesia may be of a gross degree. So far as the bodily symptoms of hysteria are concerned Freud (1894) introduced the term 'conversion' and outlined his theory in the following terms:

> In hysteria the incompatible idea is rendered innocuous by its sum of excitation being transformed into something somatic. For this I should like to propose the name conversion. The conversion may be total or partial. It proceeds along the line of the motor or sensory innervation which is related — whether intimately or more loosely — to the traumatic experience. By this means the ego succeeds in freeing itself from the contradiction with which it is confronted; but itself it has burdened itself with a mnemic symbol which finds a lodgement in consciousness, like a sort of parasite, either in the form of an unresolvable motor innervation or as a constantly recurring hallucinating sensation, and which persists until a conversion in the opposite direction takes place.

The secondary gain is the advantage which ensues from the disorder or illness and which may be directly appreciated by the patient in terms, for instance, of the avoidance of unwelcome duties or the manipulation of relationships.

Freud's 'hydrodynamic' view (Ziegler and Imboden, 1962) of the nature of 'conversion' hysteria was rather too simplistic, for the emotional distress is by no means always transmuted into the symptom; in fact, in a study of a group of patients with chronic conversion syndromes Lader and Sartorius (1968) found that anxiety, as measured both by self-ratings and autonomic activity was more pronounced than in a group of patients suffering from phobic anxiety. Nor is the affect defended against always that of anxiety; both Abse (1959) and Ziegler and Imboden have pointed out that a variety of mood patterns may predominate in these patients and depression may be as marked an anxiety. If fugue, with amnesia for personal identity, is accepted as a 'hysterical' syndrome, Stengel (1941) found a constitutional predisposition to manic-depressive psychosis in all of the 25 cases he examined and in a further paper (1943) he speculated that the fugue was in fact a symbolic suicidal act. Certainly many of the patients with such manifestations as astasia-abasia and aphonia that are seen in clinical practice today, have developed their florid symptomatology in the setting of a depressive illness.

Much has been made of the supposed indifference of the patient towards his 'conversion' symptom, the so-called *belle indifférence*; on the occasions where this is demonstrably present it is usually cited as support for the view that the primary gain has been achieved but this is a hypothetical proposition which stems from the widespread adoption of the freudian theory. Another large group of disorders, conventionally classified under the rubric of hysteria, are those disorders based upon dissociation, a temporary isolation of an area of psychic activity and resulting in various dysmnesic states. It is likely that this same psychological mechanism may explain the *belle indifférence* in those cases where it does occur. Such an explanation has been proposed by Whitlock (1967) who pointed out that if a patient is unaware, or only partially aware, of a loss of function his disability is not likely to cause him concern. Nemiah (1975) has also considered that dissociation is the basic mechanism behind all hysterical phenomena and calls in question the validity of the conventional distinction between 'conversion' and dissociative phenomena; he points out that the very use of the term 'conversion' depends upon a hypothetical construct which may in time require revision.

An alternative approach to the 'hysterical' symptom is that it represents a form of communication of distress. The phrase 'attention-seeking' is frequently used by the exasperated physician about a patient manifesting, for example, astasia-abasia and staggering and falling about in an ungainly manner; seeking attention may be just what the patient is in fact trying to do, attention and help for a disturbing disorder of mood which he finds impossible to express in words. Balint (1957) has proposed that some patients offer a symptom or an illness to the doctor in place of their emotional distress and it is indeed an important part of the art of medicine to see beyond that which is offered. According to this view 'hysterical conversion' is conceptualized as a kind of non-verbal communication couched in a protolanguage that arises in and is conditioned by the specific setting of the doctor–patient relationship' (Chodoff, 1974).

In a study of a Nigerian population Lambo (1960) found that hysteria was commoner in the urban than in the rural areas and that gross hysterical disability of a fluctuating kind was found in the rural people whereas the monosymptomatic type of hysterical reaction occurred predominantly in the sophisticated urban African. Hare (1974) has drawn attention to the changing patterns of the presentation of psychiatric disorder and a probable reason for the decline of hysterical symptomatology of the classical type (Stefanis, Markidis, and Christodoulou, 1976) is the education of doctors in psychiatry and their more perceptive attitude towards the emotional problems of their patients.

The decline of hysteria

The use of the term hysteria as a diagnostic label appears to be in decline, at least in those countries of the world with advanced medical and psychiatric health care systems. As stated in the foregoing section this decline may be partly due to a real lowering of the incidence of the classical type of symptoms; it may also in part be due to the reluctance of clinicians to use a term which is increasingly recognized, by both the public and by clinicians, to have pejorative overtones. Furthermore, the demonstration that the 'diagnosis' of hysteria is frequently in error has led to greater caution in its application even by those who defend the nosological concept.

As the use of the term declines two important studies (Slater, 1961; Slater and Glithero, 1965) have hastened this demise. In the first of these studies Slater studied 24 twin pairs (12 monozygotic and 12 dizygotic) in which the proband had received the diagnosis of hysteria; 5 MZ and 4 DZ twins were concordant for neurotic disorder but no twin had been diagnosed as hysterical. In the first degree relatives, excluding the twin, only one case of (doubtful) hysteria was found, giving an incidence for the disorder of 3 per cent, but there were 5 depressives (7 per cent), 2 epileptics, and no schizophrenics among the relatives. Comparing his findings with those of Ljungberg, Slater found himself to be in general agreement and concluded that there was no evidence for a genetic basis for the disorder called hysteria. In the second study, Slater and Glithero conducted a follow-up investigation, over a period of 7–11 years, of 99 patients who had received the diagnosis of hysteria at the National Hospital for Nervous Diseases in London. They succeeded in tracing or contacting 85 of the patients (32 men and 53 women) of whom 12 had died; in some of these patients (11 men and 13 women) an organic disorder had been recognized during the follow-up period and the diagnosis of hysteria seemed to have been based, in many of these patients, on a disproportion between the degree of disability and the physical signs, the so-called hysterical overlay of organic disease. Surveying the group as a whole, the authors were impressed by the gravity of the after-history and the frequency of diagnostic error; 8 men and 24 women (approximately 40 per cent of the sample) were not found to have developed organic disorder at the time of follow-up but even here, as Slater (1965) remarked on another occasion: 'the concept of hysteria fragments as we touch it'; for among this group of 32 patients were found 2 schizophrenics, 1 chronically anxious obsessional neurosis, and 8 patients suffering from recurrent endogenous depression. The remainder were composed of 7 patients (all young and including 2 children) who had suffered from acute psychogenic reactions with typical conversion symptoms, all of whom were well at follow-up, and 14 patients (3 men and 11 women) with more chronic states and lasting personality disorder. The authors considered that bodily disease might predispose to a state liable to be called hysteria in two major ways: a local lesion may be poorly understood (atypical facial pain and basilar artery migraine are cited as examples); alternatively, organic disease might bring about a general disturbance involving the personality and this change might then be the basis on which the hysterical symptoms develop. With respect to this latter proposition it seems likely that organic disease of the central nervous system itself is particularly likely to be the basis for the development of such symptoms (Whitlock, 1967; Slater and Roth, 1969; Merskey and Buhrich, 1975).

The work of Slater, and particularly the second study, has of course been subject to severe criticism, not least on the grounds that the sample was highly selected one, referred to a hospital for the diagnosis of neurological disease, and that a very different picture would have emerged if the sample had consisted of patients referred, say, for psychotherapeutic treatment; this criticism is justified, in so far as a much smaller proportion of the patients would subsequently be expected to develop organic disease but none the less the population would probably still fragment from a diagnostic point of view. In his Shorvon Memorial Lecture, Slater (1965) quoted the neurologist, Lord Brain:

If hysteria is regarded as a disease . . . it tends to encourage the belief that it is necessary to decide whether a patient is suffering from hysteria or from something else. But if the patient is regarded as a hysteric it allows the possibility that he may have other things the matter with him as well. He may be reacting hysterically to mental subnormality or depression or even . . . to anxiety. He may have hysteria and epilepsy or hysteria and some organic brain disease. On the other hand, the substantival idea of hysteria as a disorder leads to an enquiry as to what abnormality hysterics have in common which leads them to react characteristically.

Slater concluded that the substantival view, the designation of a patient as a hysteric, should be rejected but that it might be legitimate to retain the adjectival view of a symptom as being hysterical in form or causation.

At this stage in a discussion of hysteria it is usual to remind the reader that Sir Aubrey Lewis remarked in 1975 that hysteria was too useful a term to be put to death: 'The majority of psychiatrists would be hard put to it if they could no longer make a diagnosis of "hysteria" or "hysterical reaction"; and in any case a tough old word like hysteria dies very hard. It tends to outlive its obituarists.' However, nosological exile, if not execution, has been carried out in the United States where the word hysteria no longer appears in the latest revision of the diagnostic system (DSM-111) and where the syndromes previously classified under the category are now divided into a distinct class called *Dissociative disorders* and a subclass of *Somatoform disorders:conversion disorder*.

The term hysteria yet retains passionate advocates for its retention; Merskey (1979), for example, in his text of that title, not only argues for retention of hysteria as a clinical entity and also for the continued inclusion within that entity of the traditional crowd of disparate conditions: monosymptomatic hysteria; polysymptomatic hysteria (including hypochondriasis and Briquet's syndrome); hysterical elaboration of organic complaints; self-induced illness or damage such as anorexia nervosa and hospital addiction; psychotic and pseudopsychotic disorders (Ganser's syndrome, hysterical psychosis); hysterical personality; and culturally sanctioned or epidemic hysteria. By contrast Cleghorn (1969), surveying the collection of disorders thrown into the ragbag referred to hysteria as showing 'multiple manifestations of semantic confusion'.

The present status of hysteria

The present position appears to be that hysteria as a diagnosis can no longer be justified but that the term hysterical is still sanctioned, at least in Britain; even so it will continue to be a source of mis-understanding and disagreement for there is no single definition of the term which is universally accepted and it is necessary to ask every clinician who uses it in just which sense he wishes the term to be understood. Of the many concepts of 'hysteria' the idea that emotional stress is converted into symptoms, which was so widely accepted under the prestige of Freud's influence, is unlikely to be held for much longer as true for all the classical 'conversion' and 'dissociation' symptoms, although in some individuals it may be found to be the case. It is becoming widely recognized that such symptoms occur in the setting of a wide variety of organic and psychological disorders and may be regarded as a form of com-munication of distress. Symptoms of the underlying disorder may be apparent if looked for and very often this will take the form of unresolved emotional stress with symptoms of depression and anxiety. The *belle indifférence* is no longer held to be a universal accompaniment of such symptoms and, when it does occur, is more likely to be indicative of the dissociative mechanism that clearly operates in some cases. Hysteria has now become a term of oppro-brium which often signifies exasperation and rejection by the clinician and if for that reason alone, its retention in the diagnostic formulary is hard to accept. The classical dissociative and 'conver-sion' symptoms are now becoming rarer. When they do occur, suggestion may play a large part in their entrenchment and they will tend to persist under the influence of clinical bewilderment and multiple investigations.

Good treatment of the symptom consists of a calm explanation of its nature, if possible together with a demonstration that the function is still intact with the help of hypnosis, light anaesthesia, or some other procedure which enhances suggestibility; needless to say, it is essential to detect and treat the associated emotional disorder or disease process.

HYPOCHONDRIASIS

The term hypochondriasis is derived from the Greek word *chondron* meaning cartilage. The *hypochondrion* is the anatomical area of the abdomen underlying the rib cage which houses the liver, stomach, and spleen; it was believed that disturbance of these organs resulted in a mental disease, hypochondria or hypochondriasis. In the course of time the term underwent a transformation of meanings and, as with hysteria, a variety of concepts became associated with it (Kenyon, 1965). From a survey of the medical literature of the present century Stenbäck and Jalava (1961) isolated the following concepts: (a) nosophobic hypochondria (fear of disease); (b) somatic delusions associated with schizophrenia or manic-depressive psychosis; (c) hysterical hypochondria; (d) 'compensation neurosis' associated with somatic symptoms; (e) a personality disorder.

Pilowsky (1967) carried out a factor analysis of a questionnaire completed by patients who had been considered to manifest hypochondriacal features; three main factors were isolated; bodily preoccupation, fear of disease and conviction of the presence of disease with non-response to treatment. Not much importance can be attached to the third factor since two of the three items which had high loadings on it were rather general statements but the other two factors appear to be clinically meaningful. The most important senses in which the term hypochondriasis is used today, both by clinicians and the public, fall into three groups. The first is a morbid concern with health linked to a reverence for patent medicines, health farms, and other promotions of doubtful merit; the pre-occupation is with a search for abundant health, delay of ageing, and long life without necessarily a belief that the present state of health is poor. The second sense is the conviction of the actual presence of disease, or that disease is likely to be acquired and, unlike the first, is usually accompanied by anxiety. The third sense may be summed up by the phrase 'enjoyment of bad health' and such individuals pursue ill-health as a hobby, delighting in the acquisition of interesting symptoms which they regale in endless recital to anyone with the forbearance to listen.

Probably few clinicians today would agree with Gillespie (1928) that hypochondriasis is a specific nosological entity but it has achieved the status of being listed as one of the eight named categories of neurosis where it is defined in the Glossary of the 9th Revision of the *International classification of diseases*:

300.7 Hypochondriasis. A neurotic disorder in which the conspicuous features are excessive concern with one's health in general or the integrity and functioning of some part of one's body, or, less frequently, one's mind. It is usually associated with anxiety or depression.

However, a concern with somatic symptoms in the absence of organic disease to account for them may surpass the degree of a neurotic preoccupation and achieve the intensity of a delusional conviction; in such cases the hypochondriasis usually occurs in the setting of a recognized psychotic disorder although it may occur as an isolated psychopathological process. For this reason Kenyon (1976) proposed that hypochondriasis should be considered in the framework of a continuum of increasing seriousness of concern with health, beginning with an overawareness of normal bodily sensations and passing on to mild apprehension of disease, phobic concern, overvalued ideas, and finally to a delusional conviction of the presence of disease.

In 1961 Mechanic, a student of the sociological aspects of disease, proposed the term 'illness behaviour'; this concept is used to refer to the ways in which given bodily sensations or symptoms are perceived, evaluated, and acted (or not acted) upon by the individual. Illness behaviour encompasses both the attitude to ill-health, serious and not so serious, and the style of coping with illness, severe or mild. It includes consideration of whether the individual complains to others, seeking solace or reassurance or whether he regards his symptoms as a shameful weakness and keeps quiet about them; whether he regards minor bodily discomfort as signifying the presence of disease requiring attention or whether he shrugs it off as part of the normal vicissitudes of life; whether he makes liberal use of such articles as aspirin, laxatives, and first-aid plasters or whether he has a profound mistrust of all medicaments; whether the appearance of symptoms in adverse circumstances is part of the individual's repertoire of coping with stress or whether he employs alternative devices. In 1977 Mechanic summed up some of his insights into illness behaviour. The perception of illness may be learned in the context of the social and ethnic group and, during childhood, the response of others, particularly the parents, to minor bodily discomforts may establish a pattern of behaviour which endures throughout life. Illness behaviour may, however, abruptly change in the setting of personal stress or adverse circumstances of the group and individuals who experience psychological distress are more likely to complain of a given symptom than those free of distress such as anxiety or depression.

Mayou (1976) surveyed the factors which contributed to the expression by an individual of bodily discomfort or sensations in terms of illness symptoms. These were divided into predisposing and precipitating factors. Predisposing factors are the personality structure of the individual, his past experience of illness both of himself and others, his knowledge or relative ignorance about health matters, the pattern of illness behaviour in the cultural group to which he belongs, and his present social situation. Actual symptoms may be precipitated by the occurrence of a psychiatric disorder or by some stressful situation; they may follow some widespread publicity about illness; symptoms of a similar nature may be induced by witnessing the illness of another person, e.g. chest pain occurring in a daughter whose father has recently died from lung cancer; finally there is the important factor of iatrogenesis, symptoms being unwittingly produced or prolonged by such medical attitudes as overconcern or lack of specific explication or information.

Much has been written on the subject of the varying attitudes to illness and tolerance of bodily discomfort of various racial groups. There can be little doubt that the ethnic group to which the individual belongs is an important factor but it would be premature to pronounce the establishment of any factual information in this area since the studies have been carried out on different ethnic groups living in a limited geographical area e.g. Italians, Irish, and Jews in New York (Zborowski, 1952), Greeks and people of Anglo-Saxon stock in Australia (Pilowsky and Spence, 1977). There can be no way of being certain from these studies whether such racial differences are not related to some common personality feature which led to recent transmigration of the group, or whether the group are living under some undeclared but relevant stressful situation. Racial stereotypes are readily established but as subject to fallacious generalizations as are such statements as 'all Scotsmen are mean'. Pilowsky and Spence have underlined these difficulties by pointing out that the illness behaviour of a particular ethnic group must be conceptualized on two levels: true ethnic variation and the groups immigrant or other social status in the wider community.

The study *Social class and mental illness* (Hollingshead and Redlich, 1958) was conducted in the USA; the sample of patients was from a population undergoing psychiatric treatment. Rather more patients in social classes IV and V than in I, II, and III suffered from 'psychosomatic reactions' which were defined on the basis of prominent symptoms in one of six organ systems which were considered to be psychogenic in origin. So far as this slender evidence is reliable it may be concluded that somatization of emotional disturbance is more prevalent in the lower social classes.

Hypochondriasis and disorder of mood

Preoccupation with health and fear of disease are widespread attitudes in the population and are more pronounced in some people for a variety of cultural and experiential reasons. Awareness of, and concern about, bodily discomfort is more likely to occur if the individual is psychologically distressed (Mechanic, 1977) and, if a patient suffers from a mood disorder of morbid intensity, somatic symptoms may dominate the clinical picture and lead to the underlying mood disorder being overlooked or misdiagnosed. These dramatic symptoms may arise on the basis of normal bodily sensations or slight degrees of discomfort which the patient would ignore or tolerate without complaint were his mood normal. In 1963 Bradley studied the phenomenon of bodily pain occurring in relationship to depressive illness and he divided his patients into two groups according to whether the pain had preceded the onset of depression or had commenced simultaneously with it. Following successful treatment of the depression the pain was completely relieved in the second group but in the first group the pain persisted although the patient's tolerance for it greatly increased.

In a Maudsley lecture, Stengel (1965) considered the complicated relationship between pain and psychological disorder and the reality of what may be called psychogenic pain; at a later date, in another Maudsley lecture López Ibor (1972), spoke of the variety of symptom patterns which might be the presenting clinical features masking an underlying depressive state and among these are a variety of syndromes dominated by such 'physical' symptoms as pain and paraesthesia. A variety of factors are associated with the production of somatic symptoms in the setting of a disorder of mood. In depressive states the increased muscular tension and functional disturbance of the autonomic nervous system which are associated with the accompanying anxiety may be manifest in such symptoms as generalized muscular pain, localized pain, palpitations, respiratory distress, and digestive disturbances. Stengel quotes with approval the views of Engel, an American professor of medicine and psychiatry, that pain has many associations in the psychic economy, being linked to power over others as well as with the guilt over aggressive feelings towards others. Certainly, in this latter context, pain may be a symbolic expression of the severe feelings of guilt occurring in the setting of depression and the patient may even develop a delusional belief, centring on his somatic symptoms, that he has developed an incurable disease which has been sent to him as a punishment and for which there is no prospect of a cure.

In anxiety states the accompanying somatic symptoms are likewise based upon muscular tension, and disturbance of the function of the autonomic nervous system; they are aggravated by the accompanying apprehension and fear of disease or incapacity. Tyrer (1976) has retraced the ideas concerning the relationship of emotional states, and especially anxiety, to bodily symptoms. He pointed out that if the anxious individual can recognize the source of his anxiety he is less concerned by the accompanying symptoms of physiological arousal but if the cause for his anxiety was obscure to him then the somatic symptoms are more likely to be perceived as the source of the psychic discomfort rather than a manifestation of it:

> A patient with a dog phobia is fully aware of the cause of his fear and will therefore not attach much importance to his symptoms, whereas the patient who experiences an acute attack of panic while at rest may infer a somatic cause for the attack and regard his anxiety as secondary.

The tendency for abnormal mood to be partially or entirely manifest as bodily symptoms may be partly culturally determined and depend upon past experience and other factors. It is sometimes considered that such factors as low social class, immigrant status, male sex, and older age are all associated with the process of somatization of emotional distress. It is likely that in Britain, and indeed most parts of the world, older men who have grown up in a tradition that the display of emotion is unmanly and a weakness to be suppressed, are more likely to emphasize bodily rather than psychic symptoms when they become depressed. It may also be a factor that doctors are more likely to respond to somatic symptoms with concern. A study at the All-India Institute of Medical Sciences (Teja, Marang, and Aggarwal, 1971) found that the incidence of somatic symptoms and hypochondriasis in depressed patients in northern India was significantly higher than in British or southern Indian patients and they wrote:

> These differences may be a reflection of the level of cultural emancipation of the social group. In psychiatric illness symptoms which are assigned the status of an illness by the group to which the patient belongs, as also the expectancy on the part of the patient as to what the local medical men consider an illness, become important determinants in the choice of symptoms.

A study of hypochondriasis was carried out by Kreitman *et al.* (1965). They established a clinic in a general hospital and requested referrals from non-psychiatric clinicians of patients considered to be hypochondriacal. The majority of their patients had very long histories of somatic complaints and had undergone a great number of investigations, including operations, without the establishment of definitive organic disease (a process which the authors called 'an expensive odyssey'). Of the 120 patients, 20 were diagnosed as suffering from depressive illness and, of these, 6 recovered, and a further 9 showed substantial improvement with psychiatric treatment; a modest but worthwhile result in such a chronic population. Kreitman and his colleagues considered that the underlying mood disorder was frequently overlooked by non-psychiatric clinicians partly because it was frequently atypical and overshadowed by the somatic symptoms and partly because the disturbance of mood was attributed to the symptoms and not considered to be the cause of them. There is also the resistance on the part of some patients to the admission of depression or other mood disorder since such an admission may be considered by them to be tantamount to a confession of dissimulation.

Other factors in hypochondriasis

Other patients with prominent somatic symptoms do not suffer from an affective disorder but may be lonely or in other adverse social circumstances; others prolong symptoms for the interpersonal gains which they secure: attention, interest, sympathy, an excuse for failure, and so on. These individuals probably constitute the majority of hypochondriacs who visit doctors and hospitals repeatedly.

Dewsbury's (1973) phrase 'disease-claiming behaviour' best sums up both the behaviour and the underlying need to be sick. The symptoms of these patients may simulate either physical or psychiatric disorder although some patients feel more secure in surgical and general medical clinics, deny emotional disorder and look with disfavour upon a proposal for psychiatric referral; however, with the increasing acceptability of the concept of psychiatric illness it is probable that psychiatrists are also seeing this behaviour pattern more frequently and some patients concentrate entirely on offering psychic symptoms. Their behaviour is rather less bizarre than the 'hospital addicts' (to be described later) but whether there is a fundamental difference in the psychopathology or whether it is just a matter of the degree of disturbance is not yet established. Disease-claiming behaviour is a diagnostic trap both for the inexperienced and experienced clinician alike and frequently the greater the scientific acumen and therapeutic zeal of the clinician the more likely is he to be ensnared. Usually a correct formulation of the clinical state cannot be made until years have passed with many referrals, investigations, and treatments. However, having once arrived at such a formulation it should be the responsibility of one clinician to attempt to channel the behaviour into less expensive and more constructive patterns. Many doctors balk at this task, being well aware that they and their colleagues have contributed to the establishment of the pattern and aware moreover that they must take the full blast of the patient's hostility if they challenge the sickness concept too maladroitly. Unhappily, the general practitioner who is responsible for the overall medical management is often powerless to reverse the pattern, especially when the patient is equipped with sheaves of appointment cards to various hospital clinics and knows that his claim to a plethora of drugs and other treatments has the authoritative approval of half a dozen hospital departments.

Mead (1965) has put forward some excellent suggestions for the management of such patients, combining both sympathy and interest with firm management and a clear declaration of a recognition of the presence of unhappiness but the absence of disease. However, such management is only likely to be successful if the patient is seeing only one clinician regularly and if there has been a clear communication and agreement in management between all clinicians involved in the case. Frequently, a period of admission to hospital offers an opportunity for the assemblage of information, social as well as clinical, and a subsequent plan of management:

Mrs Ada B. was 45 years old when she was admitted to a psychiatric unit for the fourth time following her third overdose within five years. She was separated from an alcoholic husband; a son who was in frequent trouble for minor infringements of the law still lived with her and two married daughters tried to have as little contact with her as possible, one having moved to a distant part of the country and the husband of the other having attempted to forbid his wife to see her mother and certainly to have her in their home. Ada had previously been diagnosed as suffering from depressive illness; she had received two courses of ECT without clear benefit and had been taking three types of psychotropic drug over a long period of time. She had also received a diagnosis of idiopathic epilepsy three years previously and had been seen at various neurological clinics where she had accumulated a treatment regime of two types of anticonvulsant drugs although she had never actually been observed to have a fit by any of the neurologists. She complained of explosive headaches for which she occasionally took a drug for the alleviation of migraine and she had been thoroughly investigated for severe dyspepsia; no definite organic cause for the latter complaint had been discovered but she was taking antacid preparations on medical prescription. She had twice changed her general practitioner in four years.

The psychiatrist in charge of her care made a provisional formulation of disease-claiming behaviour. This was discussed at a meeting of the clinical team and it was agreed that the social worker would explore the attitudes of the family, all drugs would be rapidly withdrawn and the psychologist would arrange a programme with the registrar and the nursing staff in which the expression of symptoms would be ignored but any expression of interest in the hospital occupational programmes would be treated with interest and encouragement. All this was then sympathetically explained to the patient and it was pointed out that sickness could sometimes become a habit which was reinforced by the attitudes of doctors and nurses. At first the patient was hostile to this reversal of attitudes and complained loudly to the night nurses and even the domestic staff, whom she thought were not a party to the 'cold-hearted gang'; however, she found that attitudes of all the staff were quite consistent and surprisingly quickly she began to earn her 'rewards' of a visit from her daughter, a bunch of flowers sent by her son, a birthday tea party in the ward and even a drive into the country with the son-in-law whose hostile attitude had modified after he had understood the nature and purpose of the plan of management.

At no time during the period since drugs were stopped did she have a fit. Before she left hospital her general practitioner attended a staff meeting where the whole programme and future management was discussed. After discharge from in-patient care she attended the day-hospital for a few weeks, took up a part-time job and over the follow-up period of two years she began to enjoy life in a new way, family relationships improved and she paid no more visits to her general practitioner or hospitals.

The keystone to successful management of these unhappy people is clear communication between all involved and absolute consistency. It takes time and effort but not so much effort as would be expended if the task is neglected.

Syndromes associated with the concept of hypochondriasis

Accident neurosis

In 1961 a neurologist, Dr Henry Miller, delivered two Milroy Lectures before the Royal College of Physicians. In these lectures he reviewed 200 consecutive cases of head injury referred for medicolegal examination. All social strata were represented, from unskilled labourers to the peerage. Of these patients 47 suffered from 'unequivocal psychoneurotic complaints' and in a further 9 patients a depressive syndrome of endogenous pattern followed the injury. Miller grappled with the knotty problems surrounding the distinction of neurosis from malingering and concluded that true malingering in his patients was rare but that there was a gross exaggeration of complaints, in a number of his patients, head pains being described as 'terrific', 'agonizing', and so forth. He made the observation that the severity of the injury and the appearance of gross symptoms were in inverse proportion. He rejected the term hysteria as implying a particular psychodynamic causation and he also eschewed such terms as 'compensation neurosis' and 'litigation neurosis' as prejudging the issue of the aetiology.

Miller considered that such gross complaints were likely to occur when two conditions were fulfilled: that the accident was the fault of someone else (at least in the patient's estimation) and that it occurred in circumstances where financial compensation might be involved. He concluded that the disability was not consciously gain-motivated but that powerful forces were involved in its severity and prolongation: the trade union official who sought to pursue what he regarded as his member's interest, the solicitor pressing his client's case, and the indecisive doctor referring his patient for an ever-increasing number of opinions and investigations. He advised that the best management of such cases lay in decisive opinions and early settlement of financial compensation.

These publications provided a certain degree of clarification of a large social problem but there is a danger in adhering too rigidly to a view that persisting symptoms following head injury are *ipso facto* 'neurotic' in nature. Taylor (1967) also considered the nature of post-concussional symptoms and drew the conclusion that there was a true organically based syndrome; a leading article in the *British Medical Journal* (1967) pointed out that there was a fine distinction between Miller's accident neurosis and the organic psycho-syndrome, requiring great expertise in clinical judgement. In general, florid symptoms following relatively trivial injury are likely to fall into the neurotic group, but morning headache of a throbbing character accentuated by movement, and vertigo induced by change of posture, together with disturbance of memory and concentration, are 'common and undoubtedly organic sequelae of closed head injury'.

Furthermore, whether symptoms are gross and exaggerated or not, a careful psychiatric assessment should be included of any patient where there is doubt of the presence of psychiatric symptoms such as depression or post-traumatic phobic neurosis. A degree of reactive depression may be expected to follow any injury causing temporary or prolonged loss of earning power and a phobic aftermath of some degree will occur in any injury following a fall from a height or an underground explosion in all but the most phlegmatic. However, it must be assessed whether such additional disabilities are within the range of the normal or whether they are likely to lead to persisting true handicap unless treatment is instituted.

The appearance of gross hysterical symptoms of the 'conversion' type may be naïvely thought to sway the diagnosis in the direction of the neurotic rather than of the organic pattern; however, this is a fallacy and, as Slater and Roth (1969) point out, the appearance of indubitable symptoms of this type following a head injury is indicative that actual damage to the brain has occurred.

Dysmorphophobia

This cumbersome term is misleading for, as a leading article in the *British Medical Journal* (1978) pointed out, patients with this condition do not suffer from a phobia of bodily deformity; rather, they have an overvalued idea concerning some mild or even non-existent blemish. They may be convinced that their nose, their ears, their breasts, or some other part of their body is too small or too large, or they may ruminate upon some general idea rather than a specific part of their anatomy; for instance a man may be engrossed with the idea that he 'looks like a homosexual' and that others must notice this. A related disorder is the conviction that a disgusting smell is emanating from the body which must be perceptible to other people. Like all overvalued ideas these may border on the delusional or develop into frank delusions.

The condition was studied by Hay (1970) and among 17 patients he found that five suffered from schizophrenia and the rest all suffered from severe personality disorder of the sensitive and insecure type; the premorbid personalities of those patients who had developed a schizophrenic psychosis had also been marked by sensitivity and the conclusion was drawn that the disorder tended to develop on the basis of a specific personality structure. Hay gave no details concerning the source of referral of these patients but they probably had all been referred for psychiatric opinion. There is little information on the severity or outcome of the disorder in a non-psychiatric population but it is possible that transitory and mild disorder of the body-image of the dysmorphophobic type is not uncommon, especially among sensitive adolescents. However, patients with more severe degrees of the disorder are more likely to prevail upon their general practitioners to refer them to surgeons and it is therefore not surprising that patients undergoing surgery have a poor psychiatric outcome. In 1978 Connolly and Gipson reported their findings of a psychiatric examination of 86 patients who, fifteen years previously, had undergone rhinoplasty for cosmetic reasons and compared these patients with patients who had undergone facial plastic surgery following disease or a recent injury; of the 86 patients, 6 had become schizophrenic and 32 were suffering from severe neurosis which would certainly seem to point to a poor outcome although no account was available of the psychiatric status at the time of operation.

Certainly some patients with overvalued ideas concerning health later develop frank delusions and these patients are probably suffering from forms of psychosis allied to schziophrenia; the delusional psychosis centring around ideas of bodily infestation has been shown by Riding and Munro (1975) to respond to a neuroleptic drug which is also effective in the treatment of schizophrenia.

The hospital addiction syndrome

This is the term preferred by Barker (1962) for the disorder described by Asher (1951) under the eponymous term Munchausen's syndrome. Barker objected to the term for three reasons; first, because it implied a sharply delineated entity; second, because it focussed attention on one particular aspect, the pseudologia, which is entirely different from that of the stories of the original Baron von Munchausen; and third 'because it casts ridicule upon these pathetic patients whose illness drives them to undergo such prolonged and terrible sufferings'.

The condition is characterized by simulation of grave illness, such as abdominal emergencies, which leads to repeated admissions to hospitals and usually repeated investigations and operations. The patients travel from one hospital to another over periods of years and avoid readmission to the same hospital presumably for fear of being recognized. They have a deep distrust of psychiatrists and psychiatric hospitals. Barker studied seven patients who, over a mean period of 12 years had each undergone a mean number of 73 hospital admissions; one patient, a woman, had had 124 admissions traced over a 23-year period. The patients do not appear to suffer from any clearcut psychiatric disorder and no clear account of its aetiology has so far been offered. Asher proposed that the following factors may enter into its genesis:

1. A desire to be the centre of interest;
2. A grudge against doctors and hospitals satisfied by frustrating and deceiving them;
3. A desire for drugs;
4. A desire to escape from the police;
5. A desire for free board and lodging.

However, he admitted that these possible motives did not offer a complete explanation, taken singly or together, of such complex and persistent behaviour. Barker's patients did not appear to be addicted to drugs. A more recent review of the disorder has been undertaken by Reed (1978) but no further insights are offered as to its nature; all writers on the subject agree that it is not possible to keep any patient under observation for long enough to make a full assessment of the factors that cause and maintain such persistent behaviour.

The fully developed syndrome of hospital addiction is probably a rare condition. Asher considered it was a sharply demarcated disorder but Barker was less certain and considered the possibility that minor degrees of the condition existed.

References

ABSE, D. W. (1966). *Hysteria and related mental disorders.* Wright, Bristol.
ASHER, R. (1951). Munchausen's syndrome. *Lancet* i, 339–41.
BALINT, M. (1957). *The doctor, his patient and the illness.* Pitman, London.
*BARKER, J. C. (1962). The syndrome of hospital addiction (Munchausen syndrome). *J. ment. Sci.* **108**, 167–82.
*BENAIM, S., HORDER, J., and ANDERSON, J. (1973). Hysterical episode in a classroom. *Psychol. Med.* **3**, 366–73.
BRADLEY, J. J. (1963). Severe localized pain associated with the depressive syndrome. *Br. J. Psychiat.* **109**, 741–5.
BREUER, J. and FREUD, S. (1893). On the psychical mechanism of hysterical phenomena. In *The standard edition of the complete psychological works of Sigmund Freud,* Vol. 2 (ed. J. Strachey). The Hogarth Press, London.
CHODOFF, P. (1974). The diagnosis of hysteria. *Am. J. Psychiat.* **131**, 1073–8.
*—— and LYONS, H. (1958). Hysteria, the hysterical personality and hysterical conversion. *Am. J. Psychiat.* **114**, 734–40.
*CLEGHORN, R. A. (1969). Hysteria—multiple manifestations of semantic confusion. *Can. Psychiat. Ass. J.* **14**, 539–51.
CONOLLY, F. H. and GIPSON, M. (1978). Dysmorphophobia—a long-term study. *Br. J. Psychiat.* **132**, 568–70.
British Medical Journal (1967). Post-concussional syndrome. Leading article. *Br. med. J.* **iii**, 61–2.
*—— (1979). Epidemic hysteria. Leading article. *Br. med. J.* **iii**, 408–9.
DEWSBURY, A. R. (1973). Disease claiming behaviour. *J. R. Coll. gen. Practitn.* **23**, 379–83.
EYSENCK, H. J. (1960). *The structure of human personality.* Macmillan, New York; Methuen, London.
FARLEY, J., WOODRUFF, R. A., and GUZE, S. B. (1968). The prevalence of hysteria and conversion symptoms. *Br. J. Psychiat.* **114**, 1121–5.
FREUD, S. (1894). The neuropsychoses of defence. In *The standard edition of the complete psychological works,* Vol. 3 (ed. J. Strachey). The Hogarth Press, London.
GILLESPIE, R. D. (1928). Hypochondria: its definition, nosology and psychopathology. *Guy's Hosp. Rep.* **78**, 408–60.
*HARE, E. H. (1974). The changing content of psychiatric illness. *J. Psychosom. Res.* **18**, 283–9.
*HAY, G. G. (1970). Dysmorphophobia. *Br. J. Psychiat.* **116**, 399–406.
HOLLINGSHEAD, A. B. and REDLICH, F. C. (1958). *Social class and mental illness.* Wiley, New York.

INGHAM, J. G. and ROBINSON, J. O. (1964). Personality in the diagnosis of hysteria. *Br. J. Psychol.* **55**, 276–84.

JANET, P. (1907). *The major symptoms of hysteria.* Macmillan, New York.

KENYON, F. E. (1965). Hypochondriasis: a survey of some historical, clinical and social aspects. *Br. J. med. Psychol.* **38**, 117–33.

*—— (1976). Hypochondriacal states. *Br. J. Psychiat.* **129**, 1–14.

KREITMAN, N., SAINSBURY, P., PEARCE, K., and COSTAIN, W. R. (1965). Hypochondriasis and depression in out-patients at a general hospital. *Br. J. Psychiat.* **111**, 607–15.

LADER, M. and SARTORIUS, N. (1968). Anxiety in patients with hysterical conversion symptoms. *J. Neurol. Neurosurg. Psychiat.* **31**, 490–5.

LAMBO, T. A. (1960). Neuropsychiatric problems in Nigeria. *Br. med. J.* **ii**, 1696–1704.

The Lancet (1977). Briquet's syndrome. Leading article. *Lancet* **i**, 1138–9.

*—— (1978). Dysmorphophobia. Leading article. *Lancet* **ii**, 588.

LEWIS, A. (1975). The survival of hysteria. *Psychol. Med.* **5**, 9–12.

LJUNGBERG, L. (1957). Hysteria: a clinical, prognostic and genetic study. *Acta psychiat, neurol. scand.* **32** (Suppl.), 112.

*LÓPEZ IBOR, J. J. (1972). Masked depressions. *Br. J. Psychiat.* **120**, 245–58.

*MAYOU, R. (1975). The social setting of hysteria. *Br. J. Psychiat.* **127**, 466–9.

*—— (1976). The nature of bodily symptoms. *Br. J. Psychiat.* **129**, 55–60.

MEAD, B. T. (1965). The management of hypochondriacal patients. *J. Am. med. Ass.* **192**, 119–21.

MECHANIC, D. (1961). The concept of illness behaviour. *J. chron. Dis.* **15**, 189–94.

*—— (1977). Illness behaviour, social adaptation and the management of illness. *J. nerv. ment. Dis.* **165**, 79–87.

MERSKY, H. (1979). *The analysis of hysteria.* Baillière Tindall, London.

—— and BUHRICH, N. A. (1975). Hysteria and organic brain disease. *Br. J. med. Psychol.* **48**, 359–65.

MILLER, H. (1961). Accident neurosis. *Br. med. J.* **i**, 919–25.

NEHMIAH, J. C. (1975). Hysterical neurosis: conversion type. In *Comprehensive textbook of psychiatry* (ed. A. M. Freedman, H. I. Kaplan, and B. J. Sadock). Williams and Wilkins, Baltimore, Maryland.

PERLEY, M. J. and GUZE, S. B. (1962). Hysteria—the stability and usefulness of clinical criteria. *New Engl. J. Med.* **266**, 421–6.

PILOWSKY, I. (1967). Dimensions of hypochondriasis. *Br. J. Psychiat.* **113**, 89–93.

*—— and SPENCE, N. D. (1977). Ethnicity and illness behaviour. *Psychol. Med.* **7**, 447–52.

*REED, J. L. (1978). Compensation neurosis and Munchausen's syndrome. *Br. J. hosp. Med.* **19**, 314–25.

RIDING, B. E. J. and MUNRO, A. (1975). Pimozide in monosymptomatic psychosis. *Lancet* **i**, 400.

SLATER, E. (1961). Hysteria 311. *J. ment. Sci.* **107**, 359–71.

*—— (1965). The diagnosis of 'hysteria'. *Br. med. J.* **i**, 1395–9.
*—— and GLITHERO, E. (1965). A follow-up of patients diagnosed as suffering from hysteria. *J. Psychosomat. Res.* **9**, 9–13.
—— and ROTH, M. (1969). *Clinical psychiatry*, 3rd edn. Ballière, Tindall and Cassell, London.
SNAITH, R. P. (1968). Concepts of hysteria. *Br. J. Psychiat.* **114**, 1593–4.
STEFANIS, C., MARKIDIS, M., and CHRISTODOULOU, G. (1976). Observations on the evolution of hysterical symptomatology. *Br. J. Psychiat.* **128**, 269–75.
STENBÄCK, A. and JALAVA, V. (1961). Hypochondria and depression. *Acta psychiat. scand.* (Suppl. 162), 240–6.
STENGEL, E. (1941). On the aetiology of fugue states. *J. ment. Sci.* **87**, 572–99.
—— (1943). Further studies on pathological wandering. *J. ment. Sci.* **89**, 224–41.
*—— (1965). Pain and the psychiatrist. *Br. J. Psychiat.* **111**, 795–802.
TAYLOR, A. T. (1967). Post-concussional sequelae. *Br. med. J.* **iii**, 67–71.
TEJA, J. S., NARANG, R. L., and AGGARWAL, A. K. (1971). Depression across cultures. *Br. J. Psychiat.* **119**, 253–60.
TYRER, P. (1976). *The role of bodily feelings in anxiety*. Oxford University Press.
WHITLOCK, F. A. (1967). The aetiology of hysteria. *Acta psychiat. scand.* **43**, 144–62.
WOODRUFF, R. A. (1967). Hysteria: an evaluation of objective diagnostic criteria by the study of women with chronic medical illness. *Br. J. Psychiat.* **114**, 1115–19.
WORLD HEALTH ORGANIZATION (1978). *Mental disorders: glossary and guide to their classification with the 9th revision of the International Classification of Diseases*. Geneva.
VEITH, I. (1965). *Hysteria: the history of a disease*. Phoenix Books, Chicago.
ZBOROWSKI, M. (1952). Cultural components in response to pain. *J. Soc. Issues* **8**, 16–30.
ZIEGLER, F. J. and IMBODEN, J. B. (1962). Contemporary conversion reactons: a conceptual model. *Archs gen. Psychiat.* **6**, 279–87.
———— and MEYER, E. (1960). Contemporary conversion reactions: a clinical study. *Am. J. Psychiat.* **116**, 901–10.

5

Anorexia nervosa

THE syndrome of anorexia nervosa was described and so named by Sir William Gull in 1873 and at about the same time an independent description of the disorder was made by Lasègue, a professor of clinical medicine at the Faculty of Medicine in Paris. Morgan (1977) has traced the history of earlier reports on fasting girls and it is probable that descriptions of anorexia nervosa appeared over two centuries before those of Gull and Lasègue. In recent decades an extensive literature on the condition has accumulated and its perusal leads to the conclusion that anorexia nervosa is an enigma. Authoritative opinions have been given about the nature of the condition and in many instances these are based upon a prolonged study of the disorder; but the conclusions of different authorities are frequently in conflict and it is probable that disagreement arises from unrecognized bias in the definition of anorexia nervosa and the description of its characteristics. For example, one authority states unequivocally that anorexia never occurs in poor people (Bruch, 1978) whereas another states that all social classes are represented (Kay and Leigh, 1954); such a disparity most probably stems from bias arising from referral sources of the group of patients studied. Even an attempt to review the state of knowledge will be coloured by the preconceptions of the reviewer and it should be stated that, in the present attempt, no particular view of the nature of anorexia nervosa is adopted and it is believed that nothing certain is known about its cause, its course, or the most effective management.

Some authorities, such as Russell (1970) support the view that anorexia nervosa is a discrete nosological entity having little overlap with other organic or psychiatric conditions; others, such as Kay and Leigh (1954), have concluded that there is a wide overlap and little evidence for the view of a discrete psychopathology. It is probable that the term is used to cover a variety of disorders. Bruch (1966) considered that there were two distinct types; in the first, the patients are engaged in a struggle with an overwhelming sense of their ineffectiveness and are not primarily concerned about eating although bizarre food habits develop in the course of the disorder; the second type is less clearly defined but the primary concern is with food intake which is used in a variety of symbolic ways. King (1963) distinguished primary from secondary anorexia nervosa; in the primary form the subject finds the act of eating to be unpleasant and, despite difficulties, persists in abstention from food for the positive pleasure it affords; in the secondary form there is considered to be no primary aversion to food but abstinence is endured for the sake of some greater motive. A differentiation based upon symptomatology has been proposed by Beumont, George, and Smart (1976); patients who vomited and abused laxatives and diuretics ('vomiters and purgers') were distinguished from those who used diet control alone as a means of weight control ('dieters'). The 'dieters' were found to be intense, introverted, socially withdrawn individuals whose anorectic behaviour had started in response to stress; 'vomiters and purgers' were more extraverted, most of them had previously been obese and since simply abstention from food did not achieve the desired thinness they resorted to the other devices in addition to dieting. 'Dieters' were found to have a better prognosis.

Fries (1974) has described four patterns of disordered behaviour relating to restriction of food intake: (a) dieting for cosmetic reasons; (b) neurotic fixation on dieting; (c) anorectic behaviour; (d) anorexia nervosa. Neurotic fixation is defined as dieting behaviour which appears to be unjustified with regard to the initial and current weight; there is an anxious and fastidious concern with food intake and personal rules and restrictions are rigidly followed but weight loss is not extreme and the individual is considered to have 'retained insight'. The anorectic attitude is typified by neurotic concern with dieting as defined above but, in addition, there is a profound change of attitude with a disruption of normal eating patterns, a stubborn resistance to food intake and an atmosphere of quarrels and fuss about food and eating; episodic overeating, with vomiting and purging, may be associated with anorectic behaviour. For the delineation of 'true' anorexia nervosa he uses the criteria of loss of insight, strong denial of disturbance (however conspicuous this may be to others), a distorted perception of bodily configuration, and extreme weight loss. Fries admits that there is a degree of overlap between these patterns of behaviour and moreover that their differentiation may depend upon such an uncertain factor as the emotional rapport between the investigator and the subject but he remains confident that the patient with true anorexia nervosa is not confused with the other patterns of disturbed eating behaviour. However, other classifiers may be less certain of their ability to delineate the point on the continuum which distinguishes anorexia nervosa from the anorectic attitude especially when they are advised to deal with such notions prone to subjective distortion as 'loss of insight'; furthermore, it is accepted by most authors that anorexia nervosa may be preceded by a period of apparently normal and justified dieting and that amenorrhoea may precede weight loss. It is therefore likely that the present uncertainties about prevalence, causes, and course of the disorder may arise partly from the breadth of definition of the inclusion criteria accepted as necessary for diagnosis of anorexia nervosa.

THE SYMPTOMATOLOGY OF ANOREXIA NERVOSA

Bearing in mind the considerable variation in the clinical presentation of the disorder there are certain features which may be regarded as central whereas others are secondary to the process of starvation and others are variable associated features.

Central to the definition of anorexia nervosa is a distinct abnormality of attitude which Bruch has called 'the pursuit of thinness'. This attitude is characterized by an overwhelming fear of loss of control over body weight and a compulsive need to restrict food intake so that weight is eventually lost to a degree which cannot be rationally justified and may be life threatening, death occurring in a proportion of patients. The second central feature of anorexia nervosa depends upon an endocrine disorder which in females will be manifested as amenorrhoea. The argument that the amenorrhoea is secondary to the weight loss is difficult to substantiate since it may occur before the onset of eating difficulties (Morgan and Russell, 1975) and weight loss (Beck and Brøchner-Mortensen, 1954) and may persist for a long time after weight is restored to normal. Many authorities consider that a perceptual disturbance of the body image is a central feature and Bruch (1962) wrote of this disturbance being of 'delusional proportions'. However, recent investigators (Button, Fransella, and Slade, 1977; Garfinkel, Molodofsky, and Gardner, 1979; Strober *et al.*, 1979) have shown that this is not a constant feature and at present it should be regarded as an associated, rather than a central symptom, of the disorder.

Other features of anorexia nervosa are probably secondary to the nutritional deficiency; these are the bradycardia, hypotension, growth of lanugo, hair, dry skin, ankle oedema, acrocyanosis, reduced basal metabolic rate, hypokalaemia, hypothermia, hypercholesterolaemia, impaired regulation of water balance, and hypoplastic anaemia (*British Medical Journal*, 1971). However, it is possible that the high serum level of cholesterol is due to the abnormality of the diet rather than nutritional deficiency and the hypokalaemia is aggravated by the loss of potassium caused by vomiting and excessive purgation which are more pronounced features in some patients than in others. The hypothermia resulting from disturbed body temperature regulation may also be due not to the nutritional deficiency but to a primary disturbance of hypothalamic function (Wakeling and Russell, 1970).

Associated features of anorexia nervosa are those which may be intermittently present during the course of the disease or present in some patients and not in others. In this respect the status of perceptual distortion of body size and of vomiting and purging versus food restriction have already been considered. The other associated features are: reduction of sexual activity, overactivity, episodic overeating, and emotional disturbances.

Reduction of sexual activity is a frequent but not a constant feature of anorexia nervosa but it is sometimes considered to be a central feature especially by those who regard anorexia nervosa as a coping device adopted by the individual to thwart sexual maturation. It is sometimes observed that a low sexual drive is a common premorbid characteristic and it is possible to consider this either as a premonitory symptom of the disorder or as a basic constitutional or acquired neurotic state which plays a major part in the precipitation of the disorder.

A marked degree of strenuous activity is a feature of some patients with anorexia nervosa; vigorous bodily exercises are pursued and the patient may take to walking several miles to school or office and home again. This overactivity is part of the weight reduction programme and it is astonishing how much energy can be expended on such a low caloric intake.

Bulimia (episodic overeating) is an intermittent feature of the disorder but in some patients it is a more prominent and persistent feature; Russell (1979) has described a variation of the syndrome in which bulimia is prominent but other features of anorexia nervosa are also present which justifies the concept of 'bulimia nervosa' as a variety of anorexia nervosa. Some of these patients eat vast amounts of food in secret and induce vomiting immediately after the orgy. In common with the usual clinical picture of anorexia nervosa, bulimic patients are concerned that their weight should not rise above a self-imposed low threshold but by contrast they tend to be heavier, more active sexually, more likely to menstruate regularly and they remain fertile. Russell noted that depressive symptoms were often severe and that there was a high risk of suicide; the marked potassium loss from the repetitive vomiting added a further life-threatening hazard. Marked bulimia may follow a period of ordinary anorexia nervosa and the association with severe depression suggests that it is best regarded as an obsessional symptom supervening in the course of the disease but, as with many obsessional disorders, relief of the depression does not always lead to a cessation of the obsession; Russell noted that although depression was relieved in seven of his patients after treatment with antidepressants or ECT, bulimia continued in all of them.

The supposed 'loss of insight' is a refusal of the patients to admit to themselves or to others the abnormal nature of their eating behaviour; the drive to lose weight may be so overwhelming that all rational consideration of the effect of the behaviour is suppressed. It is often considered that anorexia nervosa is a slow attempt at suicide (Strauss, 1956), and so it may appear, but it is unlikely that many of these patients intend or wish to die through the process of starvation; when confronted with the possibility of death most patients deny its reality.

The association of other psychiatric disorder with anorexia nervosa is common and may occur at various stages of the disorder. Kay (1953) found that depressive mood accompanied the disorder in about 50 per cent of patients, anxiety and phobias in a slightly lower proportion, and obsessional symptoms in about 20 per cent. Morgan and Russell (1975) found persistent depression in 42 per cent and obsessional symptoms in 22 per cent of their patients and Hsu, Crisp, and Harding (1979) found depression in 38 and obsessions in 22 of the 100 anorectic patients who were followed up for four to eight years after treatment. Lesser degrees of emotional disorder are almost always present and are understandable in terms of the constant and unrewarding struggle in which these patients are engaged with themselves and others. Halmi (1974b) made the interesting observation that both obsessional and depressive symptoms were more common in those patients whose weight was normal before onset of the disorder, i.e. in those patients whose anorectic behaviour did not commence as a rational response to a genuine problem of obesity.

Two major systems are offered for arriving at a diagnosis, that of Russell (1970) and that of Feighner *et al.* (1972). Russell regards the presence of three features as necessary for the diagnosis:

1. The patient's behaviour leads to a marked loss of body weight and malnutrition. The abnormal behaviour consists of a studied and purposive avoidance of foods considered to be of a 'fattening nature'. . . . Often but not invariably, the patient resorts to additional devices which ensure a loss of weight: self-induced vomiting or purgation or excessive exercise. Occasionally a patient may indulge in bouts of overeating but these are followed by vomiting or prolonged starvation.

2. There is an endocrine disorder which manifests itself clinically by cessation of menstruation in those patients who are most commonly afflicted — adolescent girls or women during the reproductive period of life. The amenorrhoea is an early symptom and may precede the onset of weight loss. . . . In male subjects the equivalent symptom is loss of sexual interest and lack of potency, but in adolescent boys it may be difficult to elicit these symptoms; in them it is desirable to establish by means of hormone assays evidence of hormonal disorder. . . . In children before puberty, it is not yet possible to demonstrate an endocrine disorder characteristic of anorexia nervosa. The diagnosis can still be made tentatively by relying on other criteria, (1) and (3), but there may remain room for uncertainty.

3. A morbid fear of becoming fat, which may be fully expressed by the patient or may be more explicit in her behaviour. To safeguard herself against what she calls 'losing control' the patient strives to remain abnormally thin. She defends her attitude by asserting that to be thin is for her right and desirable, and she often appears to be absolutely convinced of the justification of her ideas. She loses all judgement as to her requirements for food and may protest that she is eating satisfactorily; she often overestimates her body weight and sets herself a precise weight above which she dare not rise.

There are in addition, greatly varying psychopathological manifestations, especially depressive symptoms, but also obsessional, hysterical and phobic symptoms. . . . One does not need to claim that there should be a specific psychogenesis in order to delineate anorexia nervosa; at the present time this is still not possible.

The criteria of Feighner *et al.* are rather more restrictive. They are:

1. Age of onset prior to 25;
2. Anorexia with accompanying weight loss of at least 25 per cent of the original body weight;
3. A distorted, implacable attitude to eating, food, or weight that overrides hunger, admonitions, reassurance, and threats, e.g. (a) Denial of illness with a failure to recognize nutritional needs; (b) Apparent enjoyment in losing weight with overt manifestation that food refusal is a pleasurable indulgence; (c) A desired body image of extreme thinness with overt evidence that it is rewarding to the patient to achieve and maintain this state; (d) Unusual handling or hoarding of food;
4. No known medical illness that could account for the anorexia and weight loss;
5. No other known psychiatric disorder, with particular reference to primary affective disorders, schizophrenia, obsessive-compulsive and phobic neurosis (the assumption is made that food refusal alone does not qualify as an obsessional or phobic state);
6. At least two of the following: amenorrhoea, lanugo, bradycardia, periods of overactivity, bulimia, vomiting.

These criteria deny the possibility of the diagnosis if the disorder commences following the age of 25, yet Halmi (1974a) reported that 13 per cent of her sample commenced after the age of 25 and at least one reliable report has appeared of anorexia nervosa commencing after the menopause (Kellett, Trimble, and Thorley, 1976). The weight stipulation denies the possibility of making the diagnosis until the disorder is fairly well advanced. The presence of amenorrhoea in fertile women is apparently not essential to the diagnosis and the stipulation that no other psychiatric disorder should be present is an unfortunate inclusion when so many careful reports have recorded the presence of prominent psychiatric symptoms.

The criteria of Russell are to be preferred for everyday clinical practice but for certain research purposes Feighner's criteria may be preferred since, if they are present, there can be no doubt of the presence of the disorder.

THE NATURE OF ANOREXIA NERVOSA

The debate continues as to whether anorexia nervosa is primarily a psychogenic disorder or whether it is a disease with a biophysical basis but with profound, although essentially secondary consequences, on the patient's emotional state and attitudes. A second debate is concerned with the nosological status of the disorder, whether it is a discrete entity or a pattern of symptoms arising in the setting of a variety of psychiatric and organic disorders.

Gull attributed anorexia to 'a morbid state of the mind' and the characteristic onset of the disorder in adolescent girls, often in the setting of emotional upheaval, with the intransigent dieting behaviour, failure of sexual interest, denial of illness, and associated evidence of emotional instability, combine to support the view that anorexia nervosa is psychologically determined; yet the precise factors in the psychogenesis are undetermined and strong assertions are frequently expounded on the basis of personal opinion alone.

Bruch has made a prolonged study of anorexia nervosa and has concluded that the outstanding characteristic of the disorder is a 'paralysing sense of ineffectiveness' (Bruch, 1966). In her latest exposition (Bruch, 1978) she puts forward the view that, even before the onset of the anorexia, the patients have endured a feeling of inability to live up to the expectations of their families and a pervasive fear of failure. They grow up with a deficiency of self-esteem and an inability to meet the challenges and opportunities of adolescence. The development of the disorder is attributed to a disturbance in family relationships; the parent's marriage is outwardly harmonious but there are supposedly deep flaws which the patient has felt it to be her duty to cover up. She has been excessively conforming and obedient to the parental wishes to the extent of suppressing her own individuality; with the approach of maturity the parents expect the girl to be independent but they do not relinquish their demands and expectations. The patient now adopts the abnormal dieting behaviour as a desperate attempt to cope with her conflicts and her feeling of inadequacy; the frantic concern with weight loss is a distorted attempt at self-assertion: 'to do something super-special by being super-thin'. Bruch castigates psychoanalysts and behaviour therapists alike for what she regards as their failure to understand the problem; however, her own dogmatic standpoint may do more harm than good for after all there is no family without some difficulties in relationships and it is all too easy to persuade an emotionally disturbed and sick young woman to shift the blame for her suffering on to her parents and their method of bringing her up.

Conflicts between the patients and their mothers are, of course, very common but they require cautious interpretation. Crisp (1965) considers that the conflict may be a repercussion of the daughter's illness rather than its cause and Theander (1970) points out that anorexia nervosa is a disorder which generates strong reactions in both the patient and the parents which is understandable when it is considered that the mother sees the daughter rejecting food and yet so often attempting to take over control of the kitchen. Kay, Shapira, and Brandon (1967) have pointed out that disturbing aspects of family life, which are often regarded as the cause of a neurosis, may be partly due to an abnormality or personality disorder of the patient and the same constitutional factors may help to create both the family conflict and the neurosis. In their own study they stated:

> In anorexia nervosa the mother's behaviour during the patient's illness may conform to the notion of the 'nagging, dominating mother' and be regarded as a causative factor. But how does a 'normal' mother behave when her daughter seems bent on self-starvation? Where does the primary disturbance lie?

They found, in their investigation, that in about half of their sample the family relationships were so abnormal as to account for the patient's disorder but in other families no evidence of gross abnormality could be found.

Dally (1977) has examined the phenomenon of 'the scapegoat' and the traditional view that, in anorexia nervosa, the mother becomes the scapegoat. He found that a large proportion of the mothers of anorectic patients were themselves suffering from depression and pointed out that this mood change may have a profound effect on the maturation of the adolescent child. He considered that in some cases the main therapeutic effort should be directed towards the mother whilst the patient herself 'only needs fattening and chatting up'. He points out the dangers of family therapy when such scapegoating is misplaced although he noted that it is useful for the patient to choose her scapegoat and to thereby direct her aggression away from herself on to another person.

Concepts of the psychodynamics of anorexia nervosa are inevitably bound up with fear of sexual maturity. Waller, Kaufman, and Deutsch (1940) examined the myths of primitive peoples dealing with beliefs in magical impregnation and quote two patients to support their view that anorexia nervosa represents an elaborate acting out of the fantasy of being impregnated through the mouth which leads at one time to the compulsive overeating and at other times to guilt and rejection of food.

Crisp (1965) considered that the majority of his patients had a strikingly poor premorbid sexual adjustment and that a sexual experience causing alarm was almost invariably associated with the onset of the disease; however, the incidents he cites were of a fairly universal kind, likely to be experienced by most adolescent girls. Moreover, Morgan and Russell (1975) found that abnormal attitudes to sex and precipitating factors of a sexual nature occurred in only a minority of their patients and in her survey of 94 patients, which included the younger age group, Halmi (1974a) found that 45 per cent of her sample had no conflicts associated with the onset of the disorder, 36 per cent had family conflict, including separation of the patient from home, 3 per cent had occupational or school conflicts and 16 per cent had sexual conflicts regarded as associated with the onset of the disorder. Theander (1970) found no evidence for rejection of the female sexual role. In another paper, Crisp (1970) found that patients had significantly higher birth weights than their own sisters and significantly earlier menarche than control subjects (though not than their own sisters); he concluded that there might be a psychobiological basis for the development of a weight phobia and that early puberty, for which the girl was ill-prepared, led her to experience fear, disgust, or guilt about sex which initiated the reversal to a prepubertal state both in a biological and a psychological sense. However, other authors (Theander, 1970; Halmi, 1974a; Warren, 1968) have noted that anorexia nervosa may develop before the menarche.

On the whole, despite the prominent symptoms of amenorrhoea, failure of libido, and loss of female bodily contours, the evidence for a predominant psychogenesis in sexual conflict is not strong. However, there is stronger evidence that weight problems have occurred in the patients and their families before the onset of the disorder. Many authors have noted that the patients tend to be plump before the onset and that some hurtful remark about their appearance starts them off on a course of dieting (initially with approval by the family) which later becomes too vigorous and uncontrolled. Halmi (1974b) made the interesting observation that obesity prior to onset of anorexia nervosa was more common among those with a later age at onset. Kalucy, Crisp, and Harding (1977) found that 23 per cent of mothers and 20 per cent of fathers were obviously overweight and that moreover 16 per cent of fathers and 23 per cent of mothers gave an explicit history of having undergone an anorectic-like disorder during their own adolescence. It seems likely that many patients who develop anorexia nervosa are aware of having some difficulty in controlling body weight long before they develop the disorder and this may rest upon a constitutional basis; some patients are frankly obese before and after recovery from the disorder. It may be this awareness of a constitutional basis of weight regulation which causes the patient to be sensitive about her body image and leads her to adopt such draconian methods of weight control during adolescence or early adulthood. It may also partly explain reports of an increase in the prevalence of anorexia nervosa which are coming in from a variety of sources (Duddle, 1973; Crisp and Kalucy, 1976; Theander, 1970; Kendell *et al.*, 1973); the pressures on young women, at least in Western cultures, to remain slim have always been strong but today the media have both intensified this pressure and, moreover, send out conflicting and confusing messages; any five-minute period of television advertising will probably proclaim both the virtue of the 'slim line' and the desirability of fattening food in close juxtaposition.

The possibility that some, as yet undiscovered, primary disorder of hypothalamic function underlies the syndrome of anorexia nervosa requires consideration. The same area of the hypothalamus regulates feeding, sexual behaviour, and menstrual activity (Donovan, quoted by Mawson, 1974) and occasionally discrete lesions, such as tumours, in this area of the brain have been reported to produce a clinical picture very similar to anorexia nervosa (Lewin, Mattingly, and Millis, 1972; Goldney, 1978). Russell (1970) has summarized the research findings that destruction of the lateral hypothalamic area in animals leads to food and water refusal whereas destruction of the ventro-medial centres gives rise to over-eating, diminished activity, and obesity. A more extensive survey of the neural regulation of food intake has been undertaken by Mawson.

Cessation of menstruation has been observed to precede gross weight loss in some patients (Kay and Leigh, 1954) and this supports the view that the amenorrhoea is based upon a primary hypothalamic disorder and is not simply a result of starvation. The first delineation of the endocrine disturbance in anorexia nervosa was undertaken by Russell *et al.* (1965) who found that urinary gonadotrophin and oestrogen excretion was low in these patients. It now seems certain that anorexia nervosa is not caused by primary disease of the pituitary but is related to hypothalamic dysfunction. This conclusion is based upon the relatively unimpaired secretion of ACTH whilst growth hormone may even be increased; thyroid stimulating hormone and prolactin are subject to subtle defects but there is a gross failure of the pituitary gonadotrophins, luteinizing hormone (LH) and follicle stimulating hormone (FSH); however, the levels of these gonadotrophins rise under the influence of administered releasing hormone (Mortimer *et al.*, 1973) which again shows that the failure does not lie in the pituitary gland itself. The endocrine dysfunction associated with anorexia nervosa is a fast expanding area of knowledge, good recent accounts of which have been undertaken by Dally, Gomez, and Isaacs (1979) and Beaumont (1979). Isaacs, in the aforementioned review, summarizes the further evidence for hypothalamic dysfunction, in that water balance regulation and thermoregulation are disturbed and concludes that anorexia nervosa should not be thought of as a disease of the hypothalamus since the endocrine changes are reversible as weight is regained and that, while psychogenic factors are important, particularly in respect to reproductive functions, the major influence on both hypothalamic function and hormone metabolism is that of starvation itself.

An intriguing sidelight has been thrown on the nature of anorexia nervosa by the ninth documented association between the disorder and XO gonadal dysgenesis (Turner's syndrome) which was reported by Kron *et al.* (1977). Such an association is unlikely to be due to coincidence and there may be either a common biological or a common psychological vulnerability; however, if the latter is the case it cannot be due to a sexual factor in view of the failure of sexual maturation in Turner's syndrome. Both disorders are characterized by hormonal disturbances; in anorexia nervosa there are low plasma oestrogen and gonadotrophin levels but in Turner's syndrome the oestrogen level is low but, as in ovarian failure from other causes, the gonadotrophin level is high. The authors speculate that individuals with abnormal gonadotrophin/oestrogen ratios may be at risk for anorexia nervosa.

The present state of knowledge of the complex interaction between psychogenic factors, hypothalamic dysfunction, reduced food intake, and weight loss has been summarized by Russell (1977). It is firmly established that the reduced food intake and weight loss are consequent upon a mental disorder, which in turn cause the endocrine disturbance, but there is probably also a direct pathway between mental disorder and hypothalamic disturbance which bypasses the factor of weight loss, as demonstrated by the fact that amenorrhoea may follow directly upon emotional upheaval. It is probable that weight loss may itself aggravate the mental disturbance. Finally, there is the possibility of a link between a disorder in the hypothalamic control of food intake and the food refusal characteristic of anorexia nervosa and possibly also of other mental functions.

THE RELATIONSHIP OF ANOREXIA NERVOSA TO OTHER PSYCHIATRIC DISORDERS

There is no certain evidence of any basic personality structure which is common to all patients who develop anorexia nervosa although Bruch (1966) noted that parents described the early development of patients as having been free from difficulties; they were described as quiet, obedient, clean, eager to please, helpful, precociously dependable, and excelling in schoolwork. Crisp (1965) concurs with Bruch in so far as he found the premorbid personality structure to be that of a timid, reserved, 'model' child but he considered that some of the attributes described as premorbid traits, such as obsessionalism, were possibly early manifestations of the disorder. Kay (1953) could find no definite premorbid personality structure but about half of his sample had obsessional traits and personality difficulties were considered to be common. Theander (1970) found that obsessional features and emotional immaturity were prominent whilst hysterical traits, low intelligence and sociopathy were rare. Halmi (1974a), from a case-note survey, found that 64 per cent of patients had been described as anxious or nervous and 61 per cent had premorbid obsessional traits. By and large a fairly uniform personality profile emerges from the literature yet it is liable to all the distortions consequent upon retrospective accounts of personality before illness.

The suggestion that anorexia nervosa is a *forme fruste* of schizophrenia is based upon the near delusional ideas held by many patients; there have been reports of anorectic patients developing schizophrenia but familial studies (Theander, 1970; Kalucy, Crisp, and Harding, 1977) lend no support to the association. There is stronger support for the view that anorexia nervosa is a form of depressive illness and many patients display fluctuating depressive symptoms, guilt and apathy. Kalucy *et al.* found a history of manic-depressive psychosis in 14 per cent of the fathers of their sample, but none of the mothers had suffered from the psychosis. Cantwell *et al.* (1977) found that a high proportion of patients suffered from depression both before the onset of the disorder and at follow-up and that a history of affective disorder was particularly common in mothers of anorectic patients; they considered the possibility that, at least in some cases, anorexia nervosa is a variant of an affective disorder. The occurrence of pronounced obsessional symptoms in some patients, together with the obsessional quality of some of the central symptoms, especially bulimia, has led to the view that the disorder is a form of obsessional neurosis (Du Bois, 1949).

On the whole the evidence that anorexia nervosa is a discrete nosological entity is fairly strong (Russell, 1970) but the clinical impression is also strong that patients who recover from anorexia nervosa later present with other forms of mental disorder and especially affective illness. The question will remain unresolved until more careful surveys of large samples of patients over a longer period of time have been reported.

THE EPIDEMIOLOGY AND COURSE
OF ANOREXIA NERVOSA

Anorexia nervosa has generally been considered to be a fairly uncommon disorder. In so far as prevalence estimates are determined from cases attending at psychiatric clinics this may be true, but a characteristic feature of anorexia nervosa is the marked tendency of patients to deny that they are ill and therefore to avoid contact with the medical services. Furthermore, when they do come under medical supervision, it is probable that less than half of them are ever referred to psychiatrists and, as Crisp, Palmer, and Kalucy (1976) point out, many are diagnosed as epilepsy, unexplained diarrhoea and vomiting, periodic oedema, polydipsia, and amenorrhoea and it is probable that a large proportion of these patients are not referred to psychiatrists or entered into case registers with the diagnosis of anorexia nervosa. Even among those patients who are under psychiatric care the true nature of the disorder may be obscured by such symptoms as depression, obsessional behaviour, and drug dependence so that again a diagnosis of anorexia nervosa is not recorded.

Kendell *et al.* (1973) undertook a survey of the incidence of the disorder in three areas where psychiatric case registers had been established: north-east Scotland, Monroe County (in New York State), and Camberwell (in London). The first area covers the city of Aberdeen and its environs and was ethnically and culturally homogeneous (during the four-year survey period of 1966 to 1969). During the period 28 female and two male cases were recorded and the average incidence was 1·6 per 100 000 per year (the sex–age specific rate for females aged 15 to 34 was 10·8 per 100 000 per year). Monroe County contained a non-white population of a little over four per cent; during the ten-year survey period 17 female and seven male cases were recorded giving an average incidence of 0·37 per 100 000 per year (females 15–34 years, 0·8 per 100 000 per year). No case was recorded in a negro patient. Camberwell is an urban area whose inhabitants are mostly of lower middle and working class occupations; in the survey period (1965 to 1971) it was probable that about six per cent of the population were immigrants, mostly from Asia or the West Indies. During the period, eight cases (all females) were recorded, one of whom was of Asiatic Indian stock; this gave an average incidence of 0·7 per 100 000 per year (females 15–34, 4·1 per 100 000 per year). A significant finding in the Camberwell area was that five of the eight cases were in social classes I and II whereas less than ten per cent of the population belonged to those classes. The authors were careful to draw no firm conclusions from these conflicting data but it was noted that in the year-by-year analyses of the periods, case detection appeared to be rising. They also felt that they could not comment on the claim (Bruch, 1965) that anorexia nervosa is rare among negroes.

A survey of a different type was undertaken by Crisp, Palmer, and Kalucy (1976) who undertook a most thorough case detection exercise among girls in private boarding schools and state day schools. The findings of this study are very surprising. The condition was uncommon at the state day schools but at the boarding schools the overall prevalence was found to be 4·6 cases per thousand and, in the over-16 years age group, 10·5 per thousand. It is unlikely that this high prevalence is a false estimate for in boarding schools the health and dietary intake of the pupils is under close supervision and all cases detected were confirmed to be suffering from true anorexia nervosa, all having lost 30 per cent or more of their original body weight in association with the other necessary features of amenorrhoea and a pursuit of weight loss. The authors considered that their findings pointed towards a definite class bias since the more wealthy sections of the community send their daughters to fee-paying schools. However, they admitted that some girls with anorexia may be sent to such schools in the hope that it would do them good to be away from home. Moreover, there is the possibility that being sent away from home may itself be a precipitant of the disease and, in addition, girls from certain types of home background which might predispose to anorexia nervosa might be sent away to school rather than be educated at home. Finally, case detection in state day schools must inevitably be less thorough than in boarding schools. However, the findings do suggest that the disorder is very much commoner than has been supposed and it also suggests that it may be a self-limiting disorder in many cases, manifest for a period at a vulnerable age group in a relatively large number of young women, the majority of whom probably recover without any specific treatment.

It is certain that anorexia is less prevalent in males than in females and a consensus of many different estimates of the female:male ratio is about 15:1. Certainly there seems to be less likelihood of a class bias at least in males; three of the six males reported by Beumont Beardwood, and Russell (1972) were from working-class backgrounds and six of the twelve male patients described by Crisp and Toms (1972) were from Class III, IV, or V.

It should be noted that there have been very few reports of anorexia nervosa occurring in people of non-European stock. Whether this points towards the often-stated belief that the disorder is a manifestation of an affluent, overfed society or to some other explanation must at present remain an unsettled question.

The matter of the course of anorexia nervosa must depend upon the severity of the disorder in the population surveyed and it is probable that patients referred to psychiatrists have more intractable forms of the disorder than patients seen by other clinicians and individuals with anorexia nervosa who do not contact the medical services at all. Beck and Brøchner-Mortensen (1954) surveyed the follow-up studies which had been carried out over the period from 1874 to 1953 which all pointed to a rather poor prognosis. Their own series was based upon patients who had been hospitalized and for the 17 patients who were followed up for more than 10 years, 15 were well and two had not improved or relapsed; they considered that the prognosis was less favourable in those patients with severe psychiatric disorder.

Two recent outcome studies (Hsu, Crisp, and Harding, 1979; Morgan and Russell, 1975) reached broad agreement on comparable populations of patients who had been followed-up for about the same period (a minimum of four years) following referral for treatment (Hsu *et al.* study) or discharge from in-patient care (Morgan and Russell study). Thirty-one of the 100 patients in the Hsu *et al.* study had received out-patient psychotherapy alone and a further 12 patients had received no treatment; 49 patients had received in-patient treatment with a weight restorative regime and all the 41 patients in the Morgan and Russell study had undergone in-patient weight restoration. The same outcome measures were used in both studies and these were based upon five areas of function: nutritional status, menstruation, mental state, sexual adjustment, and socio-economic status. In the Hsu *et al.* study, 48 per cent had a good outcome, 30 per cent intermediate, 20 per cent poor outcome, and 2 per cent died; in the Morgan and Russell study 39 per cent had a good outcome, 27 per cent intermediate, 29 per cent a poor outcome, and 5 per cent (2/41) died. Both studies agreed that longer duration of illness, later age at onset, premorbid personality difficulties, and disturbed family relationships were all predictors of a poorer outcome. As for the clinical features of the illness, Morgan and Russell found no predictors of outcome among the individual clinical features but Hsu *et al.* found that vomiting, bulimia, and anxiety when eating in the presence of others predicted a poorer outcome. In both studies it was found that overconcern about weight persisted in a high proportion of patients, even among those whose outcome was judged to be good and about half of the patients in both studies suffered from either mood disturbance or obsessional symptoms at the time of follow-up. It is of interest that the patients in the Hsu *et al.* study who had received only out-patient treatment did rather better than those who had received in-patient treatment although this may have been partly due to the lesser severity of their illness as judged by the degree of weight loss. Moreover, those who had received no treatment at all did not do so very much worse although numbers in this group were too small to make any confident comparison.

The broad agreement between these two studies, of severely ill patients referred for psychiatric treatment and subjected to conservative treatment regimes, provides a most useful yardstick against which to measure the effects of any new therapeutic measures. Even so, it is clear that there exist so many interacting variables that all future therapeutic studies will have to be reported in tentative terms.

ASPECTS OF TREATMENT

The early case

The treatment of anorexia nervosa is generally conceded to be a difficult task and few clinicians would now agree with Hurst (1939) that, in the established case, 'A few straightforward conversations are sufficient to straighten out most tangles.' However, too grave a view of the prognosis may be adopted from experience based upon hospital, and particularly psychiatric, practice. The general practitioner should bear in mind that many patients with mild degrees of the disorder will recover spontaneously; sympathetic understanding of the fears of the patient and her family will speed this process. Many parents will have heard about the disorder and may have gained an alarming view of its prognosis but they may be assured that this is based upon studies of severe cases. On the other hand, the patient with early anorexia nervosa should never be brushed aside with facile reassurance; she should be seen once or twice a month and time must also be found for an interview with the parents.

The early interviews should focus upon her attitude to the disorder and her fears about loss of control over her body weight. These fears are not without foundation for there is probably a biological basis in the homeostatic mechanisms of weight control; many patients have been overweight before the onset of dieting (Crisp and Stonehill, 1971), frequently there are weight problems in other family members, and a few patients do indeed become obese after recovery from the disorder. The general practitioner should encourage the patient to talk about any problems in her relationship with family members and with others, sexual fears and other stressful situations; her general concept of herself should be understood. A careful note should be made of what she says she eats and it is important to record her present weight, her weight before the onset of dieting and to compare these with the mean weight for height and age of the population (see Table 1); she should be asked what weight she is aiming at or if there is a weight above which she feels she dare not rise. A record should be made about vomiting, bulimia, laxative consumption, exercise, sexual activity, and, in the female, amenorrhoea and its duration. She should be informed that she should be seen once or twice a month and her co-operation sought in this matter; she may be told that this continued contact is necessary in order to understand her problems but an *essential* part of the contract should be a recording of her weight by the practice staff at each visit.

Interviews with the parents should elicit an understanding of the family relationships and tensions. The mother, whose daughter is refusing the meals she cooks for her and instead seeks to control the culinary arrangements of the rest of the family, will certainly be perplexed, irritable, or depressed; she will feel that it is somehow her impossible duty to persuade her daughter to eat properly and will feel guilty at her failure to do this. Her husband may be totally out of sympathy with the whole situation, regarding it as a nonsensical mother-daughter conflict which has nothing to do with him, and he may fail to offer the necessary understanding and support to both of them in their trial. The general practitioner should explain that the disorder is often mild and transitory and that attempts to get the patient to eat more than she feels she can tolerate will certainly fail and only serve to aggravate tension.

Referral for specialist care should be made on the following grounds:

1. A progressive fall of weight to below 15 per cent of the matched population mean weight;

2. Severe family friction so that a period of removal from the home for in-patient care is in everyone's interest;

3. Severe vomiting and purging with the attendant danger of hypokalaemia;

4. Persisting evidence of associated psychiatric disorder, especially depression;

5. A request by the patient herself for more intensive help. This is more likely to happen if the early management has been along the lines advised and she does not regard referral to hospital as a threat.

The severe case

The foregoing principles of management also apply if the patient is being seen in a medical, gynaecological, or psychiatric out-patient department. Some clinicians advise immediate admission for every established case of anorexia nervosa but in mild cases this is often unnecessary and may on occasion be harmful. However, if any of the indications listed above exist, then admission for in-patient treatment should be firmly advised. The view is widely held that patients deny illness and resist admission to hospital and this is of course true, but it is important to understand her underlying fears which lead her to adopt this attitude. She may fear that all control over her diet will be removed from her and that she will have to surrender to a forced feeding regime, which may even include tube feeding, by unsympathetic staff; she may have fantasies that her horror of gross obesity will be realized. She will be relieved to know that all these fears are understood by the hospital staff and that she will be required to play an active part in her own recovery, that her fears will be taken into account and her co-operation sought in achieving an agreed weight. She may be assured that this weight increase will stop well short of obesity and perhaps a little short of the matched population mean weight. However, she should also understand that some degree of firmness is necessary and that if fairly early and steady weight increase is not achieved then closer supervision will be necessary. Persistent vomiters may be informed of the very real health danger of this behaviour and advised, from the outset, that part of the programme of help will include restriction of

Table 1: *Desirable weights of adults according to height and frame*

| Height without shoes | | | Desirable weight in kilograms and pounds (in indoor clothing), ages 25 and over | | | | | |
| | | | Small frame | | Medium frame | | Large frame | |
metres	ft	in	kg	lb	kg	lb	kg	lb
					Men			
1·550	5	1	50·8–54·4	112–120	53·5–58·5	118–129	57·2–64	126–141
1·575	5	2	52·2–55·8	115–123	54·9–60·3	121–133	58·5–65·3	129–144
1·600	5	3	53·5–57·2	118–126	56·2–61·7	124–136	59·9–67·1	132–148
1·625	5	4	54·9–58·5	121–129	57·6–63	127–139	61·2–68·9	135–152
1·650	5	5	56·2–60·3	124–133	59 –64·9	130–143	62·6–70·8	138–156
1·675	5	6	58·1–62·1	128–137	60·8–66·7	134–147	64·4–73	142–161
1·700	5	7	59·9–64	132–141	62·6–68·9	138–152	66·7–75·3	147–166
1·725	5	8	61·7–65·8	136–145	64·4–70·8	142–156	68·5–77·1	151–170
1·750	5	9	63·5–68	140–150	66·2–72·6	146–160	70·3–78·9	155–174
1·775	5	10	65·3–69·9	144–154	68 –74·8	150–165	72·1–81·2	159–179
1·800	5	11	67·1–71·7	148–158	69·9–77·1	154–170	74·4–83·5	164–184
1·825	6	0	68·9–73·5	152–162	71·7–79·4	158–175	76·2–85·7	168–189
1·850	6	1	70·8–75·7	156–167	73·5–81·6	162–180	78·5–88	173–194
1·875	6	2	72·6–77·6	160–171	75·7–83·5	167–185	80·7–90·3	178–199
1·900	6	3	74·4–79·4	164–175	78·1–86·2	172–190	82·7–92·5	182–204
					Women			
1.425	4	8	41·7–44·5	92–98	43·5–48·5	96–107	47·2–54	104–119
1·450	4	9	42·6–45·8	94–101	44·5–49·9	98–110	48·1–55·3	106–122
1·475	4	10	43·5–47·2	96–104	45·8–51·3	101–113	49·4–56·7	109–125
1·500	4	11	44·9–48·5	99–107	47·2–52·6	104–116	50·8–58·1	112–128
1·525	5	0	46·3–49·9	102–110	48·5–54	107–119	52·2–59·4	115–131
1·550	5	1	47·6–51·3	105–113	49·9–55·3	110–122	53·5–60·8	118–134
1·575	5	2	49 –52·6	108–116	51·3–57·2	113–126	54·9–62·6	121–138
1·600	5	3	50·3–54	111–119	52·6–59	116–130	56·7–64·4	125–142
1·625	5	4	51·7–55·8	114–123	54·4–61·2	120–135	58·5–66·2	129–146
1·650	5	5	53·5–57·6	118–127	56·2–63	124–139	60·3–68	133–150
1·675	5	6	55·3–59·4	122–131	58·1–64·9	128–143	62·1–69·9	137–154
1·700	5	7	57·2–61·2	126–135	59·9–66·7	132–147	64 –71·7	141–158
1·725	5	8	59 –63·5	130–140	61·7–68·5	136–151	65·8–73·9	145–163
1·750	5	9	60·8–65·3	134–144	63·5–70·3	140–155	67·6–76·2	149–168
1·775	5	10	62·6–67·1	138–148	65·3–72·1	144–159	69·4–79	153–174

Based on weights of insured persons in the United States associated with lowest mortality (*Statist. bull. Metrop. Life Insur. Co.*, 40, Nov.–Dec. 1959).

This Table and its reference appears also on p. 1457 of *Price's Textbook of the practice of Medicine*, twelfth edition (Oxford University Press). However, a modification has been made in the Table in Davidson — 1 in has been deducted from male height and 2 in from female height — so that height is now recorded as 'without shoes'.

These weights refer to adults in the age range 20–24 years. The following adjustments should be made for other age groups (based on average weights for adults in *Scientific Tables*. Documenta Geigy):

Age 15–16 males, *subtract* 10%   Age 17–19 males, *subtract* 5%   Age 25–29 males, *add* 4%
           females, *subtract* 4%   females, *subtract* 2%   females, *add* 4%

access to the toilet for an hour or two after every meal. She should also be advised that self-medication with laxatives or other drugs is strictly forbidden and that she must not attempt to procure these medicaments. She should be told that nurses and doctors will not be too busy to listen to her and that she will have a definite period of psychotherapy every week. She may be allowed to refuse food which she particularly abhors so long as her daily diet contains some carbohydrate and a caloric value of 2000 to 2500. However, if she has extreme difficulty in tolerating this much food initially she may be allowed a little time to work up to it. All these attempts to increase the patient's co-operation and compliance in treatment will be rewarded, for there is no more difficult task in psychiatric nursing than caring for a hostile, frightened and determined anorectic patient.

Admission to hospital should be immediately followed by a thorough examination and assessment of the physical state. Investigations must include an electrolyte estimation and full haematological picture, a chest X-ray, and a skull X-ray. The latter investigation will be to detect those rare cases of hypothalamic tumour and attention should be directed to anterior clinoid erosion and calcification.

Soon after the admission there should be a staff meeting to plan the management. The therapeutic programme should never be rigid and should be tailored to the needs of every anorectic patient. On the 'agenda' should be:

1. the special problems of the patient;
2. the rate of weight gain to be aimed at;
3. which member of the nursing staff should sit and talk with the patient for half an hour or so every day;
4. who should undertake the definitive psychotherapy;
5. which member of the staff should see the parents or the spouse. It is very important in the treatment of anorectic patients to decide at an early stage who is going to do what and to arrange frequent communication between the participants in the therapeutic programme.

Special problems
These will include the degree of chronicity and the patient's general attitude to admission. If she has previously been treated as an in-

patient the reasons for failure of the therapy should be reviewed. The possibility of persistent associated psychiatric disorder should be considered and thought should be given to particular neurotic difficulties such as a fear of eating in the company of others. If the patient has particular hobbies or academic pursuits, thought should be given to the possibility of these continuing whilst she is in hospital. In the case of vomiters a clear plan should be formulated as to how visits to the toilet immediately after meals will be prevented.

Diet and weight gain

Every effort should be made to decrease the patient's sense of the 'unnatural' nature of eating. Co-operation may be increased if she is allowed to exclude one or two items from her diet and for the first week or so she may be allowed to eat rather little so long as she realizes that she will be expected to eat more each week until the calorie value of the daily food intake is in the region of 2000–2500. Sometimes much larger calorie intakes are recommended but too rapid a weight increase may well have a countertherapeutic effect since the patient is not given the time she requires to adjust to her increasing body size and is more likely to carry out her determination to lose weight again once she leaves hospital. The rate of weight gain to be aimed at should be discussed with the patient; there should be no rigidity about this matter since many factors are involved such as the chronicity of the disorder, the extent of weight loss, premorbid obesity, and the presence of depression. However, to take an example, a girl whose mean weight for height and age should be 140 pounds, but who weighed 150 pounds before the onset of dieting may have lost 30 per cent of her weight over a period of eight months so that she now weighs 105 pounds; a reasonable contract would be to aim at 5 per cent less than her standard weight, i.e. 133 pounds, over a period of eight weeks which is an average increase of three pounds a week.

Nursing care

The importance of skilled nursing in anorexia nervosa is paramount. The nursing staff must combine unobtrusive but careful observation of the patient's behaviour at and immediately after meals with the task of winning her trust and co-operation. One nurse should spend at least half an hour a day with the patient and encourage her to talk about her problems and attitudes. Before long the patient may give some indication of which nurse she prefers and this wish should be heeded; there is nothing to be gained from expecting a patient to confide in a girl of her own age when she would prefer a 'mother-figure', or vice versa.

Psychotherapy

This should be carried out by a psychiatrist or clinical psychologist and should last for at least an hour each week. The development of the weight phobia should be explored and its relation in time to any particular psychotraumatic incident or ongoing stress and difficulties in relationships. She should be encouraged to indulge her morbid fantasies in the presence of the therapist so that these may be discussed and her attitudes gradually corrected. Role-play and social skills training may be helpful in some cases and Anxiety Control Training (see last chapter) or some other anxiety-reducing procedure may have a place in the programme. An essential part of the psychotherapeutic treatment will be a process of cognitive restructuring of the patient's concept of her self, of her relationship to others, and of the consequences of the omission or performance of certain activities. Bruch has deplored the process of 'giving insight' in psychotherapy as she considers it is only likely to increase the patient's sense of her own futility. Indeed it has certain obvious dangers if carried out from any rigid theoretical view about the nature of anorexia nervosa; for instance, a therapist who adheres strongly to the belief that the disorder represents a retreat from sexual maturity may spend much time in discussing the patient's sexual problems and attempting to interpret her disorder in accordance with this view. If he is wrong (and there is no proof of the general validity of the theory although it may apply to some cases) the patient will become perplexed and lose confidence in the therapeutic process; she will be even more convinced that no one can understand her strange dilemma. The therapist must also beware of joining with the patient in some 'scapegoating' process and agreeing for instance, that her illness is all the fault of her mother. Since nothing for certain is known about the psychodynamics of anorexia nervosa, the therapist will be most effective if he confines himself to listening to, and understanding, his patient's particular problems. At a certain stage it may be of value to hold joint sessions with the patient and her family but this should not be undertaken too soon and certainly not until there is sound information about the family's problems and attitudes.

Behaviour therapy has, of course, its advocates (Agras *et al*., 1974; Bhanji, 1974) but it is unlikely that behaviour therapy alone will ever be the definitive treatment for anorexia nervosa. Nevertheless, there may be occasions when such techniques as rewards contingent upon weight gain may be incorporated into the therapeutic programme.

Contact with relatives
This should be undertaken at an early stage; the psychiatric social worker is usually chosen for this part of the therapeutic programme but it is important that he is chosen, not just because he is the social worker, but because he has a good knowledge of the problems of anorectic patients and their families. If his knowledge of this matter is inadequate it is better that a more experienced person should take on the task. The attempt should be made to see both parents at some stage but a long initial interview with the mother alone will be of considerable value. The main purpose of the contact with the relatives should be to understand their problems and attitudes to the patient and to report these back to the therapeutic team. As the time for the discharge of the patient from hospital approaches the parents will need guidance on their attitudes to the patient's food intake. They should be advised to avoid overconcern and to treat the matter of meals as naturally as possible. If there has, in the past, been a great deal of talk about diets, weight, and food, these subjects should be firmly excluded from conversation in the future.

Drug therapy
A number of different drugs have been proposed for the treatment of anorexia nervosa but so far the value of none of them is proven. Since the publication of the paper by Dally and Sargant (1960), chlorpromazine has its fervent adherents but no carefully controlled trials have established its effectiveness and it is not without its dangerous effects. Quite apart from the general neurotoxic effects of the drug it may increase the liability to hypotension, epileptic fits, and hypothermia to all of which anorectic patients are already prone. Williams (1977) has questioned the use of chlorpromazine on physiological grounds since the hormonal disturbance of the disease is associated with hyperprolactinaemia and this may be induced by chlorpromazine itself; he considers that persisting amenorrhoea after weight has returned to normal may be partly caused by

continued treatment with chlorpromazine. Another drug which has gained some popularity is the antihistamine, cyproheptadine; one recent blind trial (Goldberg *et al.*, 1979) has suggested the effectiveness of this drug but further confirmation is required before this can be accepted.

Other drugs which have been proposed for the treatment of anorexia nervosa on theoretical grounds are L-dopa (Mawson, 1974) and bromocriptine (Harrower, 1979). These are interesting suggestions which await evaluation. Antidepressant drugs are only of value if there is an associated persistent affective disorder.

Summary

The management of anorexia nervosa is an undertaking which calls for good team work and allowance for the considerable variation between patients. There may be occasions when vigorous therapy is not to be advised and Crisp (1967) has pointed out the danger of suicide if such a course is undertaken in patients whose disorder is of over ten years' duration. There are no facts available concerning the relapse rate in relation to the rapidity of weight gain in a hospital refeeding regime but it is probable that patients who gain weight too rapidly will lose weight again once they leave hospital, and for this reason the calorie content of the diet recommended here is lower than that generally advised; for instance a leading article (*Lancet*, 1979) recommended a diet of 3000–5000 calories but this is probably far beyond the patient's tolerance. Many clinicians who have had considerable experience in the treatment of anorexia nervosa have recorded the occasional spontaneous recovery of patients with long-standing illness and Sir William Gull, who gave the disorder its name, may also be allowed the last word:

> As regards prognosis none of these cases, however exhausted, are really hopeless while life exists; and for the most part the prognosis may be considered favourable.

References

AGRAS, W. S., BARLOW, D. H., CHAPIN, H. N., ABEL, G. G., and LEITENBERG, H. (1974). Behaviour modification of anorexia nervosa. *Archs gen. Psychiat.* **30**, 279–86.

BECK, J. C. and BRØCHNER-MORTENSEN, K. (1954). Observations on the prognosis of anorexia nervosa. *Acta med. scand.* **149**, 409–30.

*BEUMONT, P. J. V. (1979). The endocrinology of psychiatry. In *Recent advances in clinical psychiatry* (ed. K. Granville-Grossman). Churchill Livingstone, Edinburgh.

—— BEARDWOOD, C. J., and RUSSELL, G. F. M. (1972). The occurrence of the syndrome of anorexia nervosa in male subjects. *Psychol. Med.* **2**, 216–31.

*—— GEORGE, G. C. W., and SMART, D. E. (1976). 'Dieters' and 'vomiters and purgers' in anorexia nervosa. *Psychol. Med.* **6**, 617–22.

BHANJI, S. and THOMPSON, J. (1974). Operant conditioning in the treatment of anorexia nervosa : a review and retrospective study of eleven cases. *Br. J. Psychiat.* **124**, 166–72.

British Medical Journal (1971). Anorexia nervosa. Leading article. *Br. med. J.* **iv**, 183–4.

BRUCH, H. (1962). Perceptual and conceptual disturbances in anorexia nervosa. *Psychosomat. Med.* **24**, 187–94.

—— (1966). Anorexia nervosa and its differential diagnosis. *J. nerv. ment. Dis.* **141**, 555–66.

—— (1978). *The golden cage: the enigma of anorexia nervosa.* Open Books, London.

BUTTON, E. J., FRANSELLA, F., and SLADE, P. D. (1977). A reappraisal of body perception disturbance in anorexia nervosa. *Psychol. Med.* **7**, 235–43.

CANTWELL, D. P., STURZENBERGER, S., BURROUGHS, J., SALKIN, G., and GREEN, J. K. (1977). Anorexia nervosa: an affective disorder? *Archs gen. Psychiat.* **34**, 1087–93.

CRISP, A. H. (1965). Clinical and therapeutic aspects of anorexia nervosa, a study of thirty cases. *J. Psychosomat. Res.* **9**, 67–78.

*—— (1967). Anorexia nervosa. *Br. J. hosp. Med.* **1**, 713–18.

—— (1970). Reported birth weights and growth rates in anorexia nervosa. *J. Psychosomat. Res.* **14**, 23–50.

—— and KALUCY, R. (1974). Aspects of the perceptual disorder in anorexia nervosa. *Br. J. Med. Psychol.* **47**, 349–61.

—— and STONEHILL, E. (1971). The relationship between aspects of nutritional disturbance and menstrual activity in anorexia nervosa. *Br. med. J.* **iii**, 149–51.

*—— and TOMS, D. A. (1972). Primary anorexia nervosa or weight phobia in the male: report on 13 cases. *Br. med. J.* **ii**, 334–8.

—— PALMER, R. L., and KALUCY, R. S. (1976). How common is anorexia nervosa? A prevalence study. *Br. J. Psychiat.* **128**, 549–54.

*DALLY, P. J. (1977). Anorexia nervosa: do we need a scapegoat? *Proc. R. Soc. Med.* **70**, 470–4.

—— and SARGANT, W. (1960). A new treatment of anorexia nervosa. *Br. med. J.* **i**, 1770–3.

—— GOMEZ, J., and ISAACS, A. J. (1979). *Anorexia nervosa.* Heinemann, London.

Du BOIS, F. S. (1949). Compulsion neurosis with cachexia (anorexia nervosa). *Am. J. Psychiat.* **106**, 107–15.

DUDDLE, M. (1973). An increase of anorexia nervosa in a university population. *Br. J. Psychiat.* **123**, 711–12.

FEIGHNER, J. P., ROBINS, E., GUZE, S. B., WOODRUFF, R. A., WINOKUR, G., and MUNOZ, R. (1972). Diagnostic criteria for use in psychiatric research. *Archs gen. Psychiat.* **26**, 57–63.

FRIES, H. (1974). Secondary amenorrhoea, self-induced weight reduction and anorexia nervosa. *Acta psychiat. scand.* (Suppl. 248), 23–45.

GARFINKEL, P. E., MOLODOFSKY, H., and GARDNER, D. M. (1979). The stability of perceptual disturbances in anorexia nervosa. *Psychol. Med.* **9**, 703–8.

GOLDBERG, S. C., HALMI, K. A., ECKERT, E. D., CASPER, R. C., and DAVIS, J. M. (1979). Cyproheptadine in anorexia nervosa. *Br. J. Psychiat.* **134**, 67–70.

GOLDNEY, R. D. (1978). Craniopharyngioma simulating anorexia nervosa. *J. nerv. ment. Dis.* **166**, 135–8.

GULL, W. W. (1874). Apepsia hysterica. *Clin. Soc. Trans.* **7**, 22–8.

HALMI, K. A. (1974a). Anorexia nervosa: demographic and clinical features of 94 cases. *Psychosomat. Med.* **36**, 18–25.

—— (1974b). Comparison of features of patients with different ages and weights at onset of anorexia nervosa. *J. nerv. ment. Dis.* **158**, 222–5.

HARROWER, A. D. B. (1978). Bromocriptine in anorexia nervosa. *Br. J. hosp. Med.* **20**, 672–5.

*HSU, L. K. G., CRISP, A. H., and HARDING, B. (1979). Outcome of anorexia nervosa. *Lancet* i, 61–5.

HURST, A. (1939). Discussion on anorexia nervosa. *Proc. R. Soc. Med.* **32**, 744.

KALUCY, R., CRISP, A. H., and HARDING, B. (1977). A study of 56 families with anorexia nervosa. *Br. J. Med. Psychol.* **50**, 381–95.

KAY, D. W. K. (1953). Anorexia nervosa: a study in prognosis. *Proc. R. Soc. Med.* **46**, 669–74.

—— and LEIGH, D. (1954). Treatment and prognosis in anorexia nervosa. *J. ment. Sci.* **100**, 411–31.

—— SCHAPIRA, K., and BRANDON, S. (1967). Early factors in anorexia nervosa compared with non-anorexic groups. *J. Psychosomat. Res.* **11**, 133–9.

KELLETT, J. M., TRIMBLE, M., and THORLEY, A. P. (1976). Anorexia nervosa after the menopause. *Br. J. Psychiat.* **128**, 555–8.

KENDELL, R. E., HALL, D. J., HAILEY, A., and BABIGIAN, H. M. (1973). The epidemiology of anorexia nervosa. *Psychol. Med.* **3**, 200–3.

KING, A. (1963). Primary and secondary anorexia nervosa syndromes. *Br. J. Psychiat.* **109**, 470–9.

KRON, L., KATZ, J. L., GORZYNSKI, G., and WEINER, H. (1977). Anorexia nervosa and gonadal dysgenesis. *Archs gen. Psychiat.* **34**, 332–5.

The Lancet (1979). Anorexia nervosa: to investigate or to treat? Leading article. *Lancet* ii, 563–4.

LEWIN, K., MATTINGLEY, D., and MILLIS, R. R. (1972). Anorexia nervosa associated with hypothalamic tumour. *Br. med. J.* ii, 629–30.

MAWSON, A. R. (1974). Anorexia nervosa and the regulation of intake: a review. *Psychol. Med.* **4**, 289–308.

*MORGAN, H. G. (1977). Fasting girls and our attitudes toward them. *Br. med. J.* **ii**, 1652–5.

*—— and RUSSELL, G. F. M. (1975). Family background and clinical features as predictors of the long term outcome in anorexia nervosa. *Psychol. Med.* **5**, 355–71.

MORTIMER, C. H., BESSER, G. M., McNEILLY, A. S., MARSHALL, J. C., HARSOULIS, P., TUNBRIDGE, W. M. G., GOMEZ-PAN, A., and HALL, R. (1973). Luteinizing hormone and follicle stimulating hormone test in patients with hypothalamic–pituitary–gonadal dysfunction. *Br. med. J.* **iv**, 73–7.

*RUSSELL, G. F. M. (1970). Anorexia nervosa: its identity as an illness and its treatment. In *Modern trends in psychological medicine* (ed. J. H. Price). Butterworth, London.

*—— (1977). The present status of anorexia nervosa. *Psychol. Med.* **7**, 363–8.

*—— (1979). Bulimia nervosa: an ominous variant of anorexia nervosa. *Psychol. Med.* **9**, 429–48.

—— LORRAINE, J. A., BELL. E. T., and HARKNESS, R. A. (1965). Gonadotrophin and oestrogen excretion in patients with anorexia nervosa. *J. Psychosoma. Res.* **9**, 79–85.

STRAUSS, E. B. (1956). Suicide. *Br. med. J.* **ii**, 818–20

STROBER, M, GOLDENBERG, I., GREEN, J., and SAXON, J. (1979). Body image disturbance in anorexia nervosa during the acute and recuperative phase. *Psychol. Med.* **9**, 695–702.

THEANDER, S. (1970). Anorexia nervosa. *Acta psychiat. scand.* (Suppl. 214), 7–194.

WALLER, J. V., KAUFMANN, M. R., and DEUTSCH, F. (1940). Anorexia nervosa: a psychosomatic entity. *Psychosomat. Med.* **2**, 3–16.

WAKELING, A. and RUSSELL, G. F. M. (1970). Disturbances in the regulation of body temperature in anorexia nervosa. *Psychol. Med.* **1**, 30–9.

*WARREN, W. (1968). A study of anorexia nervosa in young girls. *J. Child Psychol. Psychiat.* **9**, 27–40.

WILLIAMS, P. (1977). Anorexia nervosa and the secretion of prolactin. *Br. J. Psychiat.* **131**, 69–72.

6

Sexual dysfunction

In no other area of human behaviour is there such a complex interaction between biophysical and psychosocial factors as in the mechanisms that subserve the sexual response. An understanding of these
factors is necessary if therapeutic intervention in sexual dysfunction
is to be successful. The compendious works of Kinsey, Pomeroy,
and Martin in the demographic field and of Masters and Johnson in
the physiological and clinical fields, together with a vast amount of
research in the sociological and anthropological aspects of sexual
behaviour, have done much to lighten ignorance and replace ob-
scurantist dogma, yet much is still uncertain and disputed.

Alongside the increase in scientific knowledge, there have been
profound alterations in psychosocial perspectives, especially in
those parts of the world in which people of European stock predominate; the discovery of reliable and effective methods of contraception together with a decrease in infant mortality have led to an
increasing emphasis on the pleasurable rather than the procreative
aspects of sex and groups, both small (homosexuals) and large
(women), are learning to express their views and requirements and
they are beginning to be heard with respect and understanding
rather than contempt and outrage.

ANATOMICAL AND PHYSIOLOGICAL
CONSIDERATIONS

Despite the obvious differences in the developed genitalia of males
and females there are underlying physiological functions which the
sexes have in common. Kinsey and his colleagues (*Sexual behaviour
in the human female*, p. 593) conclude: 'The anatomic structures
which are most essential to sexual response and orgasm are nearly
identical in the human male and female. The differences are relatively
few. They are associated with the different functions of the sexes in
reproductive processes but these are not of great significance in the
origins and development of sexual response and orgasm.'

Masters and Johnson have subdivided the human sexual response into the four phases of excitement, plateau, orgasm, and resolution and this has led to much clarification of thought about psychosexual dysfunction. In both the male and female the basic neural control of the sexual response is the same and consists of spinal reflexes with autonomic and somatic components subject to facilitation and inhibition by the higher nervous centres. In the spinal cord, two main centres subserve the sexual response; the first has its outflow through the second and third sacral roots and this outflow is concerned with the vasocongestive mechanisms underlying the plateau response in both sexes. The second centre has its outflow through the first and second lumbar roots and subserves the orgasmic phase. The first outflow is parasympathetic and the second is composed of sympathetic fibres.

In the male, the shaft of the penis consists of three cylindrical structures capable of distension with blood to the limits of the surrounding fascial sheath. Distension converts the flaccid urinary penis into the erect procreative phallus. A degree of conscious control may be exerted over the vasocongestive phase so that a man may produce and lose the erection alternately over a long period of time but a defect in this control leads to the clinical entity of premature ejaculation.

At a certain phase of the sexual response emission occurs; this is the secretion of seminal fluid by the prostate and seminal vesicles and at this stage ejaculation becomes inevitable and no longer under control of the will. Ejaculation is the process of powerful expulsion of the spermatic fluid and is completed in a series of spasmodic contractions of the muscles surrounding the base of the penis. After the orgasmic phase, during which ejaculation occurs, the stage of resolution is reached during which further sexual excitement is not possible; the duration of this phase varies with the sexual drive and probably also with age and may last from a few minutes to several hours. The force of the ejaculation also diminishes with age but it is rare for ejaculation to be so completely inhibited that emission alone occurs, but should this happen spermatic fluid simply seeps from the urethra instead of being forcibly expelled.

In the female, the first phase of the sexual response is associated with the secretion of fluid resulting in a moistening of the vagina. Erectile tissue is situated around the vestibule of the genital tract, the labia minora, and the lower third of the vagina. Distension of this tissue results in the orgasmic platform which grips the penetrating penis during the plateau phase. During this phase the upper part of the vagina distends into a cavity in which the seminal fluid pools. The clitoris, the sensitive tissue corresponding to the male glans, swells slightly and everts upward under its hood of skin at the anterior part of the vulva.

The orgasm which follows the plateau phase is transmitted by the clitoris and terminates in general bodily myotonia and spasmodic rhythmic contractions of the muscle surrounding the lower part of the vagina.

The hormonal basis of sexual function is an area of considerable complexity and present ignorance (Bancroft, 1977). Both oestrogen and androgens are found in males and females. In prepubertal children the levels of the hormones are low but at puberty the androgen level rises in both sexes but to a far greater extent in the male. In the female, on the other hand, the rise in oestrogen is greater. In the male, the major source of androgen supply is from the testes and, deprived of this supply by prepubertal castration, there occurs a major reduction in the development of secondary sexual characteristics, as exemplified by the harem eunuch; however, some sexual development is possible and probably dependent upon extragonadal sources of androgen. The discovery that the antiandrogen drug, cyproterone acetate, diminishes sexual drive in the male is a further pointer to the necessity of androgens for the male sexual response.

The effect of oestrogen and progesterone on female sexuality is far from clear. Neither surgical removal of the ovaries nor the menopause necessarily leads to a decline in the woman's sexual interest but the removal of both ovaries and adrenal glands does produce a definite decline in sexual arousal and this effect may depend upon the removal of all sources of androgen rather than other hormones.

There is no certain correlation between sexual interest and the cyclical changes of oestrogen and progesterone during the menstrual cycle. Subhuman mammals will receive the male only during oestrus, i.e. at the time of ovulation. For humans, the findings of Kinsey, Pomeroy, and Martin (*Sexual behaviour in the human female*, p. 610) led to the conclusion that sexual interest is greatest shortly before the menstrual period. However, more recently Udry and Morris (1968) found that rates of intercourse and orgasm were clearly related to the menstrual cycle and were much higher during mid-cycle and this finding was the same for unmarried women, who were presumably not trying to conceive, as for married women; neither of the groups was using oral contraceptives.

Whether sexual drive is partly determined by constitutional factors or is entirely dependent on psychological factors and availability of the partner is not known. It is probable that hormone levels have some relationship to sexuality. Cooper *et al.* (1970) divided a population of men presenting with potency problems into two groups, according to whether the problem was considered to arise from psychological and situational factors or whether these were relatively lacking and whose problem was to be considered as 'constitutional' in origin. Using a measure of androgen function based upon urinary excretion of testosterone they found that the constitutional group had significantly lower levels but they did not conclude that this lowered androgen level was necessarily a cause of the libidinal failure but that it might be a reflection of, rather than a cause of, the diminished sexual activity. There is some evidence for this latter view; Fox *et al.* (1972) found that plasma testosterone levels increased by as much as 25 per cent following intercourse although they did not increase following masturbation.

There is a modest decline in testosterone production as age advances (Leading article, *British Medical Journal*, 1975) and there is also a decline of male sexual activity with increasing age but it is premature to link the two events and Kinsey and his colleagues inclined to the view that the lowered sexual drive in older men was due to a decline of interest resulting from the repetition of the same act with the same partner over many years. The question remains open.

SOME PSYCHOLOGICAL CORRELATES OF SEXUAL FUNCTION

This area of enquiry is so vast that no justice can be done to it in a brief exposition such as this, and it is not possible to do more than touch upon a few topics.

The interaction between an individual's biophysical endowment for sexual activity, his innate personality structure, the effects of early and ongoing experience, and the social and sexual mores which he has imbibed, lead to an infinite variety of sexual interest and activity. It is well for any sex therapist to bear this in mind for it is commonly overlooked and even those who claim to be expert in psychosexual disorder tend to approach the subject from their own viewpoint and to judge normality by their own standards. Is it 'normal', for instance, for a girl to experience orgasm during the early phase of her marriage? The liberated women today will answer positively but Kinsey's research, conducted only 20 years ago, showed that the majority of women did not. How frequently should intercourse between a married couple take place to be considered 'normal'? Again Kinsey, Pomeroy, and Martin (*Sexual behaviour of the human male*, p. 197) found, in the American population they studied, that ejaculations (i.e. total sexual outlets, not just hetero-sexual intercourse) could vary between once in thirty years and thirty times a week throughout the whole of thirty years. These ex-treme variations are of course rare, but it is quite another matter whether even the extremes should be considered to be abnormal or pathological. The frequency of sexual outlets for Kinsey's males showed three-quarters of the population varying between one and six a week which leaves a quarter falling beyond these limits. As Kinsey and his colleagues pointed out, people at opposite poles of the frequency spectrum would be considered as very similar sorts of persons by close friends who did not know their sexual histories. The figures for the female frequency of outlet showed an even wider variation with a higher proportion in the lesser frequency range.

Kinsey and his colleagues showed that an individual's position on the continuum of strength of sexual drive was remarkably constant for that individual, showing only a gradual decline with age. Other major sources of fluctuation of sexual activity are physical and mental health, the degree to which he is preoccupied by matters other than sexual gratification, the sexual requirements of his part-ner, and the extent to which he (she) is content and secure in the relationship. Probably the advent and availability of sexually titil-lating literature and films will increase sexual activity, if only for a short period, of those who make use of the opportunity.

It is a fact to bear in mind during sexual counselling, that the person who strives for too long to attain a level of sexual activity greater than that which nature and nurture have allotted, is in for disappointment and frustration. In the sexual clinic it is not un-common to find a middle-aged man referred for 'impotence'. The history reveals that at the age of forty-five he is anxious to maintain the same sexual outlet he enjoyed at twenty-five, fearing that to re-duce the frequency would be tantamount to admitting to early senescence. Concerned about his decreasing ability to maintain his previous frequency he becomes introspective and increasingly anxious about his performance so that the way is paved for a true erectile dysfunction.

The debate continues as to the cause of decline of sexual activity with age, which may be partly due to physical and partly to psychological factors. For the 4108 men in the population they surveyed, Kinsey, Pomeroy, and Martin (*Sexual behaviour of the human male*, p. 237) found 'only stray cases of impotence' between adolescence and thirty-five years of age (in this context the term 'impotence' refers to total disinterest in sexual activity either with a partner or through solitary masturbation). At the age of fifty, 6·7 per cent of the men had become impotent and this figure rose to 27 per cent at seventy and 75 per cent at eighty years of age. Comparable figures for women are not quoted but sexual interest is maintained for at least as long as in men and it is possible, because of the lower 'need to perform' that the sexual response may be maintained, given a potent partner, into old age.

Although the experience of orgasm through masturbation is likely to be as high in women as in men during the younger age range, the woman's orgasmic response in heterosexual intercourse was, in Kinsey's study, surprisingly low (*Sexual behaviour of the human female*, p. 383). They found that only 49 per cent experienced coital orgasm during the first month of marriage but the response tended to rise as the relationship continued so that after one year 75 per cent experienced orgasm at least some of the time. By the fifteenth year of marriage there were still 10 per cent of women who never experienced orgasm during marital coitus but the investigation ended with a note of optimism by recording the case of a woman who achieved her first coital orgasm after twenty-eight years of marriage!

The extent to which Kinsey's findings in an American population in the 1940s and 1950s can be considered relevant to other cultures today awaits further research. However, if it is accepted that the orgasmic response of women in intercourse tends to increase with experience, then the reason for this increase must be sought. There can be little doubt that a part of the variation is due to anxiety about the relationship and its stability. Fears of pregnancy and the expectation of pain, concern about the transgression of social mores, and the continuing psychological effect of early strictures against sexual activity and its association with pleasure as opposed to guilt, all probably play a part. In both sexes anxiety is a potent inhibitor of sexual performance and it may be that the more knowledgeable and liberated young women of today are less prone to orgasmic failure than their mothers and older sisters. Facts, however, are few. In a British survey of young adults (Schofield, 1973) 376 men and women were asked about sexual problems. Over half (57 per cent) replied that they had such a problem and some mentioned more than one. Of all the problems mentioned the most frequently reported was that of anxiety over sexual performance which was a matter of concern for 21 per cent of men and 13 per cent of women.

Another survey of sexual habits carried out in England (Gorer, 1971) failed to agree with Kinsey's conclusion that sexual activity declined consistently from puberty onwards, and pointed out that the Kinsey survey was concerned with all 'outlets' (masturbation being the most important) whereas the British survey was concerned with heterosexual intercourse alone. Gorer concluded that high rates of marital intercourse were correlated with earlier puberty, a higher educational standard, and greater financial prosperity and considered the belief that the working class was more sexually active than the middle class was a myth promoted by a few novelists, mostly themselves of middle-class origin. That survey also concluded that younger married people in Britain were less tormented by neurotic fears of sexual inadequacy which seemed to be widespread in some other societies and this conclusion seems to be at variance with the findings, just quoted, of Schofield. It is clear that whilst meaningful data can only be collected by population surveys, such surveys are at the same time very hard to conduct and liable to pitfall and error.

For men the commonest source for anxiety was the capability to maintain erection for long enough to complete a satisfactory intercourse. So strong is the man's psychological investment in this ability that a single failure, even after a long period of potency, may lead to repetitive anxious concern and prolonged or permanent potency problems. A woman's emotional problems with sexuality are frequently of a different nature to simple concern about adequacy of performance. Guilt about sex may be more deeply rooted in childhood admonition and precept. Masters and Johnson (1970) stated that the young girl or woman has to struggle with psychosocial enigmas, cultural restrictions, and her own physical sexual awareness. However, the situation may be changing, and perhaps quite rapidly, as a result of modification of public attitudes, more explicit sexual activity on television, safer contraception, and possibly better education in schools. Gwynne Jones (1974) wrote: 'If we are in a time of sexual revolution, it is in relation to female sexuality. Of course, sex embraces far more for a woman than a man, it includes all functions related to pregnancy and childbirth. Not so long ago, social attitudes in our culture attempted to restrict their interest to these functions. Women were not expected to enjoy sexual intercourse but to submit to it passively as a duty to their husbands. They were even thought to be incapable of orgasms.' However, the major differences in emphasis in attitudes to the sexes today is stated by the same author: 'The psychosexual development of girls deviates from that of boys at puberty, the dramatic event for them being the onset of menstruation. In adolescence in our culture, and unlike boys, girls tend to be more concerned with acquiring role behaviour related to marriage than with genital sex. Fewer girls masturbate than boys and less frequently, and masturbation quite often follows, instead of precedes, an interpersonally induced orgasm. Social sanctions against girls' sexuality are stronger than against boys' but girls are actually encouraged to view boys as potential husbands. Unlike boys they are well versed in the concept of romantic love and enter into highly charged emotional relationships. The romantic path is the more likely to lead to sexual arousal, no doubt a fact quite well known to Casanova.'

It is usually thought, and stated, that in coitus the woman is slower to reach orgasm than the man. This may well be true of a proportion of women and these may predominate in the clinic but Kinsey, Pomeroy, and Martin (*Sexual behaviour of the human female*, p. 688) found no evidence that this was true for most women. Their work did however confirm what had been recognized for centuries, that fantasy plays a less important role in the sexual life of women than of men. Portrayals of nude figures, genitalia, and sexual activity caused significantly less erotic arousal in women than in men. Fantasies during masturbation were less important for women than for men and only through moving pictures, romantic literature, and being bitten did women in the survey admit to erotic arousal equivalent to that of men. Kinsey and his colleagues remark than men find it difficult to understand why women are not aroused or even interested in the type of material which they show to them in the hope of providing sexual arousal. The women, on the other hand were equally unable to comprehend why their men, given satisfactory sexual relations in the home, should need to seek additional portrayals of sexual stimulation. However, Kinsey and his colleagues, as always, warn of the tremendous range of variation and in women the range in this area is greater than men; a few women in the survey admitted to the experience of orgasm through fantasy alone which 'almost never happens among the males'.

Most writers on sexual technique, including Masters and Johnson and Kaplan (1974), express the view that the man requires less emotional investment in the partner in order to attain sexual satisfaction; the trade of prostitution certainly attests to this. However, the reverse may be true for women. Masters and Johnson considered that, for many women one of the most frequent causes for orgasmic dysfunction, either primary or situational, is lack of love and respect for the marital partner.

Kaplan deals in a detailed way with the many psychological determinants, immediate and remote, of sexual dysfunction. Among the immediate causes are fears of failure often exacerbated by pressure to perform; overconcern about pleasing the partner and a rooted fear of rejection; an inability of the couple to communicate about guilt and defensiveness and about erotic feelings; and inadequate sexual techniques. The remoter causes spring from early childhood experience and precept which may have equated sex with sin and with punishment. She also quotes Harlow's famous experiment in which monkeys, deprived of affectionate physical contact in infancy, had later difficulty in forming sexual relationships.

Among the many influences on sexual ability and satisfaction arising from the dyadic relationship, she mentions such important conflicts, overt or concealed, as power struggles, dependency needs, egotistical assertion, punishment, anger, and unrecognized sexual sabotage by the partners, one of the other.

It is clear that competent sex therapy cannot be based upon any one narrow theoretical concept and cannot be successful without a wide knowledge of the person and his partner.

PHYSICAL DISORDER AND THE SEXUAL RESPONSE

Whilst the majority of people who come for advice to a psychosexual clinic suffer from no physical disorder sufficient to account for the sexual dysfunction, it is, none the less, true that many believe, and indeed wish to believe, that there may be a physical explanation for their difficulty. Many people will not accept the clinician's assurance that the condition is psychogenic unless a physical examination has been carried out and at an early stage this should be done. It is futile and frustrating for all concerned to attempt to treat, by psychotherapy, a young man whose erectile difficulty arises from phimosis or a young woman whose vaginismus really is based upon a tight hymen. The clinician should therefore keep in mind the physical disorders that may result in sexual dysfunction. A useful summary appears in the work of Helen Kaplan, *The new sex therapy*.

Congenital lesions

There are a number of relatively uncommon congenital disorders such as hypospadias, undescended testicles, and vaginal atresia. The effect of undescended testicles need not result in sexual dysfunction but the man will probably be sterile. In this connection castration, either deliberate or through disease (e.g. mumps orchitis) or injury, need not lead to deficiency of sexual arousal or performance. However, if testicular development is congenitally deficient or fails early in life there is likely to be some diminution of normal sexual drive and administration of testosterone may produce improvement in the individual's sexual performance. In the post-pubertal male testicular loss is likely to have a psychological rather than a physical effect upon the man's sexual function.

The matter of the relation of testosterone to sexuality is a complicated one, partly because the testes are not the sole source of androgen. Probably, if adrenal glands were ever removed along with the testes, total libidinal failure would ensue as it does in women subjected to both bilateral oöphorectomy and adrenalectomy.

Local genital disease

A few conditions will cause interference with sexuality through mechanical interference or associated pain. In the male, a tight foreskin (phimosis) and associated infection (balanitis) are not uncommon and should always be excluded. Surgical correction is a simple matter. A curious condition of unexplained cause is Peyronie's disease. In this condition fibrous cords develop in the penis and lead to the characteristic description of upward bowing of the penis during erection which may make penetration difficult. Other commoner disorders which lead to difficulty in intercourse on occasion are swellings such as hydrocoele and hernia. They are more likely to lead to sexual difficulty if the man's libido or interest in his partner is already waning or if his concern about the disorder has become exaggerated through neurotic factors. Inflammatory conditions (urethritis, cystitis, and so on) will of course embarrass intercourse through pain so long as the condition remains untreated.

Prostatectomy does not usually affect the man's sexual response, unless libido was already failing, but weakness of the bladder neck may lead to loss of ejaculate through reflux into the bladder and this may cause acute concern with adverse effects upon total sexual function unless the condition is properly explained to the man.

In women there are many local causes for dyspareunia (painful intercourse) including local cysts and caruncles, infections of the genital, urinary and pelvic organs, endometriosis, broad ligament tears, and so on. Clitoral adhesion is a diagnosis in and out of fashion but there is a female equivalent of male phimosis which, according to Kaplan, is an extremely rare condition. Women may be reassured that hysterectomy will not of itself, lead to lowered sexual function. Vaginal repair operations occasionally cause difficulty if the resulting vaginal outlet is too small.

Other systemic disease will impair sexual arousal in both sexes through general malaise. There are not many diseases which specifically affect sexual function although the list of 'endocrine causes of impotence' given by Cooper (1972) includes acromegaly, Addison's disease, adrenal neoplasms (with or without Cushing's disease), castration, chromophobe adenoma, craniopharyngioma, diabetes mellitus, eunuchoidism (including Klinefelter's syndrome), feminizing interstitial-cell tumour, infantilism, ingestion of female hormones and antiandrogen substances, myxoedema, obesity, and thyrotoxicosis. Kaplan includes hypothyroidism but not thyrotoxicosis as a cause of lowered libido. Recently, interest has been roused in a disorder of pituitary function which produces hyperprolactinaemia and associated sexual dysfunction, clinical evidence of hypogonadism, and lowered testesterone concentrations. This may represent a rare form of disorder presenting with sexual dysfunction but routine screening by measurement of prolactin concentration in all men with sexual dysfunction, unless there is also evidence of hypogonadism, is not indicated (Leading article, *British Medical Journal;* 1978).

Of this list, the only disorder which must always be considered in a psychosexual clinic is diabetes mellitus. Since sexual dysfunction may be a presenting symptom of the condition, Masters and Johnson advise routine exclusion of the disorder in all people attending a psychosexual clinic. There is an undoubted and common association between diabetes and sexual dysfunction in both males and females. (Kolodny, 1971; Kolodny *et al.*, 1974; Rubin and Babbott, 1958; Ellenberg, 1971; Faerman *et al.*, 1974). It is probable that the dysfunction is based upon local neuritis in men and probably also in women although in women the exact mechanism is in greater doubt. Kolodny and his colleagues come to the interesting conclusion that, in the male, the onset of sexual dysfunction is not related to the duration of diabetes whereas in the female there is a strong correlation between orgasmic failure and the duration of diabetes. The discovery of diabetes in a person presenting with a sexual problem (or alternatively the onset of a sexual dysfunction in a known diabetic) presents a clinical problem calling for skill and discernment. It has been pointed out that the sexual failure in diabetes is never total and that moreover, libido is not necessarily affected. The presence of morning erections in the male strongly suggests that the dysfunction is psychogenic and not organic. The paper by Renshaw (1975) should be studied by any therapist having to deal with the problem. Therapeutic despair should *not* be betrayed, certainly to a couple whose mutual sex interest is still high.

Of the neurological disorders it is said that sexual dysfunction may be a presenting symptom of multiple sclerosis. Alarm should not be raised about that issue unless there is at least some other evidence of the disease. The relation of sexual dysfunction to spinal cord injury has been most studied in the male (Munro, Horne, and Paull, 1948; Talbot, 1949; Zeitlin, Cottrell, and Lloyd, 1957; Bors and Comarr, 1960; Silver, 1975; Silver and Owens, 1975). The man with injury to the spinal cord is usually capable of having erections although this will be less likely if injury to the sacral segments and cauda equina had occurred. The possibility of retention of ejaculatory function is less likely. Sexual counselling to the spinal disabled calls for a high degree of both neurological and psychological competence.

The association between sexuality and disorders of the brain is complex as might be expected. The association between temporal lobe epilepsy and sexuality is usually reported as a diminished drive (Hierons and Saunders, 1966; Johnson, 1965) but the reverse may occur. Lennox and Lennox (1960) in their major work on epilepsy cite a case of a woman with overabundant sexuality (nymphomaniac) who was found to have a tumour in the temporoparietal region of the brain.

Drugs and the sexual response

Many drugs may have effects upon sexuality. In a few cases these are well documented and the effect could be predicted from pharmacological knowledge but in others the evidence of an interference with the sexual response is vague and inconclusive. It is possible that a patient may attribute a pre-existing dysfunction to the effect of a drug more recently prescribed. Alarm about the presence of a disease which warrants the prescription of a drug may induce anxiety about sexual activity, with consequent dysfunction, which again may be wrongly attributed to the effect of the drug. In many cases it may be difficult to determine to what degree a sexual dysfunction is a true drug effect or merely thought to be so by the patient.

In no case is this uncertainty greater than in the use of those synthetic hormones used for contraceptive purposes. In some women there may be an enhancement of sexuality which may be related to the greater security of risk against unwanted pregnancy whilst in others, alarm about reported side effects or a prevalent belief that depression and loss of libido are inevitable accompaniments of contraception by the 'pill', may lead to these adverse effects. There is in fact little real evidence that the various oestrogens and progestogens of these contraceptives produce a true libidinal lowering or depressant effect, and the complicated area of research is well surveyed by Weissman and Slaby (1973).

All hypnotics, narcotics, sedatives, and tranquillizers are likely to produce a general lowering of sexual drive through their intrinsic effect upon general arousal. Such an effect may be welcome to those who do not wish to engage in a sexual relationship. Common sense will inform most people that sexuality will be diminished after taking a hypnotic drug but there may be less certainty about the effect of the sedative drugs such as benzodiazepines which are currently widely prescribed for every minor ill and emotional problem. These drugs too, taken in chronic dosage, will lower the sexual drive but occasionally, by diminishing anxiety, they may actually improve performance although their effect in this direction is likely to be short-lived as tolerance develops. There is no rational ground for prescription of these drugs on any basis apart from occasional dosage when increased anxiety is anticipated. Many people are helped by the advice to stop the drugs.

Drugs with peripheral effects upon the autonomic nervous system may be expected to have some effect upon the sexual response, particularly in the male. Drugs which produce sympathetic blockade may interfere with ejaculation whereas drugs with anticholinergic effects may interfere with erection. Some drugs used in the treatment of hypertension will therefore produce ejaculatory difficulties through their postganglionic effect and such drugs are guanethidine and bethanidine. Other drugs used in the treatment of hypertension do not have such an effect although it is claimed that diminished sexuality results from central sedation. This is often stated about the drug alpha methyldopa but Bulpitt and Dollery (1973) found no evidence of such an effect. Other drugs with anticholinergic action such as propantheline bromide and many antiparkinsonian drugs may be expected to interfere with erectile capacity.

Many of the major groups of drugs used in the treatment of severe psychiatric illness have autonomic effects. The problem of the management of severe depressive illness and consequent loss of libido with drugs such as tricyclic antidepressants, which themselves may occasionally interfere with sexual response, is a matter requiring careful clinical judgement. Sometimes such drugs have been advocated for the direct treatment of sexual dysfunction. For instance the neuroleptic drug thioridazine has been claimed to have a beneficial effect in premature ejaculation and if this is the case it is presumably the antiadrenergic rather than the anticholinergic effect which is operative although the general sedative effect of the drug may also play some part by decreasing anxiety.

One drug in the butyrophenone group, benperidol, is claimed to suppress sexual drive in those with deviant sexual behaviour. Kaplan states that another member of this group, haloperidol, has an antilibidinal effect and it is therefore possible that such an effect is a general property of this group of drugs. It is more certain that cyproterone acetate does exert a true antiandrogen effect and so directly suppresses sexual drive. Segraves (1977) has summarized the evidence implicating various drugs in disturbances of the sexual response.

A SCHEME FOR EXAMINATION

A formulation of the sexual difficulty of a person or couple must rest upon a thorough assessment of the immediate problem, with its recent and more remote origins, the effect of the problem upon the person or the relationship, and the attitudes of the person and the partner towards the problem. Competent sex therapy can only proceed on the basis of a full formulation of the difficulties; no mere 'diagnosis' will suffice. Erectile dysfunction is an extremely common presentation of sexual and personal difficulties, but there is a world of difference between erectile dysfunction occurring for the first time in a depressed middle-aged man with a harmonious marriage and erectile dysfunction in a young man with a basically homosexual orientation trying desperately to abide by social and familial pressures to establish a heterosexual relationship. To date much research in the field of sexual dysfunction is largely meaningless because of the prevailing habit of defining the population merely by a diagnostic label.

To arrive at a useful formulation of a psychosexual problem requires both experience and tact. There will be a tendency on the part of the patient to suppress certain information which may be of great importance and the facts about which need to be delicately but firmly established. The clinician must be aware that the patient may also overemphasize certain events because he thinks them to be important. In no other area of practice is it so necessary for the clinician to be able to put the patient at ease, to be at ease himself and to be able to inject a little humour into the proceeding whilst sensing and deeply respecting his patient's difficulties in expressing thoughts and attitudes which he may never before have had to put into words. It is important to avoid the impression of conducting a rigid interrogation according to a fixed plan and yet to be certain of acquiring all the information he needs in order to construct a useful formulation on which to base a plan of treatment. He will certainly fail in this task unless he has in mind a clear scheme of the information he must obtain.

Before proceeding with the examination there are some important considerations.

The first of these is a matter of joint or separate examination if the couple arrive together. The view is sometimes held that sex is a mutual involvement and that both partners *must* be interviewed together from the commencement. This is not my view; on the contrary I am convinced that, unless the couple are given the opportunity of a separate interview initially, then the clinician can never be sure he is in possession of the whole truth. There are some people who just will not, cannot, and should not be expected to reveal sensitive details such as infidelity and homosexual inclination in front of their partner, at any rate at their first session. If the separate interview is undertaken then the patient (or his partner) must be assured that no information which he divulges to the clinician will be related to the partner except with his prior consent. If, and only if, this assurance is given can the clinician feel that he might arrive at most of the truth. Having given the assurance the clinician must, of course, be scrupulous to adhere to it.

Sometimes the couple may come to the clinic together. The clinician will have some indication of who is 'the patient' (the doctor's referring letter will usually indicate this). If such is the case 'the patient' will be called into the clinic room and then, if both come forward together they may be informed that it is the usual clinic practice to see people separately in the first instance. If they then state that it is their wish to be seen together from the start, then of course their wish should be granted. If they do come together, but one is seen separately, then the presence of the other partner should be acknowledged by a brief separate or joint interview at the end of the session. It is a profound mistake to send away a partner, who has been sufficiently concerned to attend; not only may this be hurtful to the partner but a valuable opportunity to increase knowledge of the situation will be lost.

Another very important initial consideration is the matter of confidentiality. Notes of a psychosexual clinic should be kept separate from other hospital or clinic notes and filing cabinets containing them should be kept locked. Patients should be assured, that although notes will be made, these will *not* find their way into general hospital files where they may be open to inspection by a large number of people. Patients may not worry, or even have thought of this issue at the time but years later the matter may become one of acute concern (e.g. a teenage daughter becomes employed as a filing clerk at the local general hospital). The person may then recall and rest upon the assurance that was given that psychosexual clinic notes were kept separately from other notes. Hastings (1963) has this to say: 'I would rather risk forgetting important

details of a person's intimate life than risk someone else reading or
hearing what the patient had said.'

Two fundamental points must be kept in mind throughout the
examination and at the end of the session the clinician should have
definite information in respect to both these points. They are:

> 1. Is the dysfunction primary or secondary? In other words
> has it always existed or was there a time when the patient had a
> more normal or satisfactory sexual ability?
> 2. Is the dysfunction only manifest in one particular situation
> and not in others or with one partner and not with others?

For instance, a man may complain of erectile dysfunction with his
wife who is his only sexual partner. Careful elicitation of the facts
during the examination revealed that on a few occasions, when away
from home on holiday, he had achieved a satisfactory intercourse; a
further enquiry revealed that the dysfunction had commenced at a
time when his mother came to live with them and slept in a bedroom
separated from their own by a wall which was anything but sound-
proof.

During the examination the following broad areas of information
should be touched upon (but in each individual some will be more
relevant than others):

> 1. Early family life. Acquisition of sexual information.
> 2. Development of personality and specifically of attitudes
> towards sex. Sexual orientation and particular deviation.
> Fantasies.
> 3. Sexual experience prior to present partner.
> 4. Sexual experience with present partner. Attitudes of
> present partner to dysfunction. Sexual dysfunction in partner.
> General relationship with partner. Pregnancy and birth control.
> 5. Any specific precipitant of dysfunction.
> 6. Medical history. Psychiatric history. Current drug treat-
> ment. Alcohol consumption.
> 7. Present mental state.

The examination is not complete and a formulation cannot be made
without information in all these areas and the development of detailed information in some of them.

Family life and acquisition of sexual information

The early development of concepts about sex and sexual relationships occur during childhood and may be enduring. The earliest model on which the individual may base a concept of relationships is usually that of his parents' behaviour to each other. Factual sexual information may have been easily acquired or the subject may have been shrouded in misinformation and enveloped with attitudes of guilt and taboo. The recollection of preparedness for, and reaction to, first menstruation or first ejaculation may be revealing.

Developing adolescent attitudes to the opposite sex may have been free and uninhibited or the reverse. At this stage the person may have become aware of frank heterosexual aversion or homophile inclination which may have been temporary or persistent. A persistent deviation, such as paedophilia, may have its roots in early infantile and adolescent sexual fears and guilt.

The development of personality may profoundly affect future sexual attitudes and adjustment. For example, marked shyness will lead to difficulties in forming new relationships and overabundant self-centredness will lead to callous neglect of the needs and satisfactions of others. The tendency to indulge in reverie, sexual fantasy, and romantic dreams may help the person prepare for a real sexual encounter but, on the other hand, carried too far, it may lead to problems in the attempt to establish a satisfactory relationship.

The art of eliciting sexual deviance and variance in orientation requires to be studied for many people tend to deny the attraction of any attitude they consider 'kinky' or 'queer'. The subject should be gently introduced and the wording should suggest that the clinician considers such attitudes to be general and acceptable rather than the exception to be rejected. A suitable introductory phrase may be: 'Most people pass through a phase of attraction to their own sex and, for some, this remains as strong or even stronger than attraction to the opposite sex. How would you say you rate yourself on this matter?' 'Some people find they are only "turned on", that is fully aroused sexually if some object is present or some fantasy is present in the mind; you've probably heard of the term fetishism and the common examples such as rubber or silk probably occur to you. Would you say on careful reflection that there are any such objects that commonly turn you on, or on the other hand are there situations which do the reverse, i.e. turn you off sex?'

Prior sexual experience

This may or may not be of significance. It will be of obvious importance if the first attempt at a sexual relationship led to derisive failure and persistent feelings of inadequacy or guilt about sex. There may be other aspects of earlier sexual encounters which lead to enduring attitudes which are relevant to the patient's later dysfunction.

Confidence and competence in an earlier relationship, with sexual failure in the present one, would point to some feature of the present relationship as being at the root of the difficulty. If the sexual dysfunction commenced a long time before attendance at the clinic it is important to discover in just what circumstances it began and whether, if there had been previous sexual competence, the onset was gradual or sudden following some specific event.

Relationship to present partner

An overall picture of the relationship of the patient to the partner should be gained. Later this will be supplemented and modified when the partner is seen either alone or together with the patient. Before enquiry is made for details of the sexual relationship it is important to know whether the couple love and respect each other, whether they really wish their relationship to endure, and whether they enjoy each other's company. Past and present infidelity of both partners should be ascertained. It is not infrequent that in therapy a wife of a man with sexual dysfunction will express her misgivings about his fidelity to her. The therapist must have a fair idea as to whether the accusations are realistic or not before he can handle the interview correctly.

It is necessary to ascertain the sexual relationship of the couple before the onset of the dysfunction if it commenced during their relationship, and then careful enquiry should be made as to the mode of onset of the difficulty. It is very important to know about the partner's attitude to the dysfunction and the willingness to be involved in a therapeutic programme if this should be advised. The therapist has a difficult task ahead if a woman with orgasmic dysfunction comes for help and then reveals that her husband is totally disinterested in her lack of sexual pleasure and has informed her that she is at liberty to try to 'get herself sorted out' so long as he does not have to go to the clinic too. It is essential to gain an impression as to whether the partner him- (or her-) self has a sexual dysfunction and whether this pre-existed or is secondary to the other's difficulty (some husbands of women with vaginismus, for instance, have marked potency problems and the marriage was based upon a form of assortative mating).

It must be established whether there are particular aspects of the partner's behaviour or technique of making love which upset or 'turn off' the patient. For instance, a woman may have had long-standing fears of being smothered or suffocated, but had kept this to herself, and her husband had always taken the superior position during intercourse. On the first occasion that she was allowed to take the superior position she experienced an orgasm. It is important to know whether the dysfunction is total or partial, constant or inter-mittent. For instance does a man with erectile dysfunction prevent-ing intercourse ever experience an erection — during sleep, during masturbation or on waking in the morning? Can the woman with orgasmic dysfunction be aroused to a climax during mutual or solitary masturbation? Attitudes to pregnancy and methods of birth control should be known. Fear of further pregnancy may be an overriding factor in the dysfunction or a man with premature ejaculation may be increasing his sexual anxiety whilst fumbling to fit on a condom.

A history of a specific precipitant of the dysfunction should not be missed as its presence may have great importance in the formula-tion and in planning an approach to therapy.

The medical history

This may or may not have relevance. It is more common for a dys-function to be ascribed to an episode of disease than the reverse. None the less the presence or history of some physical disorders may be of relevance. For instance, diabetes mellitus may be leading to sexual difficulty through neurogenic mechanisms or a vaginal dis-charge may have aroused fears of a venereal infection which had never been fully resolved. Certain statements or descriptions by the patient may arouse suspicion of a condition such as Peyronie's disease.

A past history of mental illness may be important. Loss of libido is symptomatic of a depressive illness as well as other psychiatric disorders. Not infrequently the failure of sexual response persists after recovery from the depression. Psychosexual dysfunction may be the presenting disorder in a depressive state and other symptoms of the depressive illness may be masked or muted. It is of major importance not to miss the presence of a depressive illness for the approach to therapy will be quite different from that of most sexual dysfunction. *Conjoint marital counselling will be a waste of time and utterly frustrating for all concerned so long as one partner remains in an untreated depressive state.*

A careful drug history is required for a full formulation of any psychosexual disorder, and the part played by alcohol consumption in the precipitation or continuation of the dysfunction should be firmly established.

THE PATTERNS OF SEXUAL DYSFUNCTION

The common-or-garden words impotence and frigidity should now be replaced by more descriptive and meaningful terms. Only in this way can confusion be avoided, communication be improved, and advance be made in knowledge of psychosexual disorders. Moreover, the old terms have acquired pejorative and derogatory overtones which are quite out of place in a psychosexual clinic. The term 'frigid' for instance has been taken into lay parlance to indicate that the woman not only has a sexual problem but that she is an aloof, defensive, and perhaps self-centred person, whereas the woman coming to the clinic with vaginismus or orgasmic dysfunction may have none of these adverse traits. That the term 'impotence' will persist has been partially ensured by Masters and Johnson's use of it in *Human sexual inadequacy.*

The classification of sexual dysfunction produced by Masters and Johnson is:

For the male:
   1. Impotence: (a) primary, (b) secondary;
   2. Premature ejaculation;
   3. Ejaculatory incompetence.
For the female:
   1. Orgasmic dysfunction: (a) primary, (b) secondary;
   2. Vaginismus.

Dyspareunia is also included in their classification and many of the causes of painful intercourse are listed.

The definitions of 'primary' and 'secondary' differ, according to Masters and Johnson, between the sexes. A man is to be regarded as suffering from 'primary impotence' if he has never been able to achieve penetration either in heterosexual or homosexual intercourse but they recognize that such a primarily impotent man may yet have experienced orgasm through solitary or mutual masturbation. The woman is defined as suffering from primary orgasmic dysfunction only if she has never, throughout her entire life, experienced orgasm.

The classification scheme of Kaplan is an improvement and is as follows:

  1. Inhibition of the vaso-congestive phase;
        Men: erectile dysfunction
        Women: general sexual dysfunction
  2. Inhibition of, or failure of control over, the orgasmic phase;
        Men: premature ejaculation
                retarded ejaculation
        Women: orgasmic dysfunction (Kaplan uses the term 'orgastic')
  3. Vaginismus (no equivalent in the male).

Much the same definitions of primary and secondary forms of erectile dysfunction and orgasmic dysfunction as those produced by Masters and Johnson are followed. It is stressed that erectile dysfunction, orgasmic dysfunction, and general sexual dysfunction may all be markedly situational or they may be total; in the latter case change of circumstances under which intercourse is attempted or change of partners does not alter the defective sexual response. Kaplan's major innovation is the separation of orgasmic dysfunction from deficiency of arousal in the woman, although she admits that there is usually an overlap of the conditions. General sexual dysfunction is the condition in which the woman derives little if any erotic pleasure from stimulation in the sexual context. In orgasmic dysfunction the woman can enjoy the physical intimacy of sexual intercourse but she consistently fails to experience orgasm. Both these disorders may be primary or secondary, situational or total in origin.

Both Masters and Johnson's and Kaplan's classificatory systems are deficient in one major respect and advances in therapy will depend on a clear recognition of the matter. This is the failure to consider the constitutional as opposed to the psychogenic varieties of both male and female dysfunction. In the present day climate of enthusiasm for psychotherapeutic treatment for sexual dysfunction, it is perhaps unfashionable to consider that erectile dysfunction or general sexual and orgasmic dysfunction is not always induced primarily through psychological mechanisms. Among authors who have recognized that constitutional factors may play a major part in the manifestation of some forms of erectile dysfunction have been Johnson (1965) and Cooper *et al.* (1970). Ansari (1975) classified a population of 65 men with erectile dysfunction as follows:

> Group 1. (21 cases) Subjects in this group had an acute onset triggered off by psychological or physical trauma.
>
> Group 2. (23 cases) This group had an insidious onset linked with long-term psychological or physical trauma.
>
> Group 3. (21 cases) This group had insidious onset without any discernible psychological or physical factors.

In a post-treatment follow-up study (Ansari, 1976) it was found that the prognosis in the third group was the poorest, whether the management had been by conjoint marital counselling, by supportive psychotherapy combined with tranquillizers, or by no treatment other than interview. The scheme of Cooper and his colleagues (1970) for determining the relative importance of 'psychogenic' or 'constitutional' factors in men with potency problems has already been given (see p. 175). Their finding that men with the 'constitutional' pattern of dysfunction had significantly lower androgen levels than the 'psychogenic' group has so far not been confirmed but the strong possibility does exist that for some men there is a biophysical cause for their dysfunction. If this is true for men, it may also be the case for some women with orgasmic dysfunction.

Erectile dysfunction

In this condition there is a failure to obtain or maintain penile erection long enough for coital penetration of the partner. It may be primary or secondary, it may be situational or total and the underlying libidinal drive may vary from weak or absent to strong. In the case of a weak libidinal drive this may be longstanding and possibly regarded as a trait of individual, or libidinal failure may have occurred more recently. In some men with erectile dysfunction penetration can be achieved, but the erection then fails and intercourse cannot be completed although sometimes, on withdrawal, the erection is again produced and the couple can proceed to mutual gratification through masturbation.

An occasional erectile failure is probably a very common experience and the question may arise as to how often this might occur to be abnormal. Masters and Johnson classify a man as secondarily 'impotent' if he has erectile failure during at least 25 per cent of his sexual opportunities. However, no such figure can be meaningful and the decision for management by simple reassurance, or by more lengthy treatment, must be based upon a full formulation of the problem.

Erectile failure is a common honeymoon experience for the couple who have not previously engaged in intercourse; it is usually easily overcome, so that only the more persistent cases will appear in a psychosexual clinic. A single failure to maintain an erection may be a particularly psychotraumatic event for some men, especially for those who have not previously experienced the difficulty and who have a high personal investment in their sexual capability. For this reason, subsequent anxiety over future sexual intercourse is likely to be high and failure may be repetitive. It is for this reason that a history of prolonged erectile dysfunction so often commences with a sudden onset.

Premature ejaculation

Ejaculation may occur before vaginal entry and by any definition this is premature. It is more problematic to state a period of time after penetration, short of which the condition of premature ejaculation may be said to occur. It is only possible to say that premature ejaculation occurs when both partners agree that the man ejaculates too quickly. Even so, some people have unreasonable expectations of the duration of coitus. Cooper (1969) puts the matter thus: 'In this respect, Kinsey *et al.* have pointed out how feelings of sexual inadequacy and a belief of prematurity (unwarranted in reality) may develop and become fixed, because the male fails to live up to a popular sexual stereotype (usually a sexual superman) that men can sustain erections and continue coitus for hours on end. It is clearly necessary to establish whether the condition exists in fact, or only in the mind.' There may, therefore, be occasions on which, after full consideration the clinician will advise the couple that they do not really have a sexual dysfunction. Kaplan considers that the experience of mutual orgasm is relatively unusual and nothing but anxiety will be generated in striving to obtain it. However, for the majority of couples who come to a psychosexual clinic with supposed premature ejaculation, the problem is real enough.

Most writers on the subject point out that the premature ejaculator is generally an anxious man. However, this is by no means the rule. Premature ejaculation, like other forms of sexual dysfunction may be primary or secondary, situational or total, but it is probably less prone to alteration with changing circumstances or partners than erectile dysfunction. Schapiro (1943), in a review of over a thousand cases, considered that in about half his patients premature ejaculation ensued after a period of normal function and that these patients showed symptoms such as insomnia, fatigue, and circulatory and digestive disorders. The other half had prematurity from the very first attempt at coitus, there was a familial history of the disorder, libido was high, and other neurotic symptoms were not marked. Cooper (1969) has partly confirmed this finding.

Retarded ejaculation

Kaplan's term is to be preferred to Masters and Johnson's 'ejaculatory incompetence' or the Latin *impotentia ejaculandi*. However, even that term is misleading, for the fully developed dysfunction is characterized by a complete absence of intravaginal ejaculation even though erection remains strong. People do not usually seek help for this dysfunction unless the ability to ejaculate is complete and therefore the term 'absent ejaculation' may be more accurate than 'retarded ejaculation'.

Masters and Johnson considered the disorder to be relatively rare. They described, in their cases, a universal background of sexual repression and an attitude of dislike of their wives and of women generally. (Reading their account of these men, one is surprised to learn that Masters and Johnson 'cured' 14 out of the 17 cases referred to them.) they considered the dysfunction to be usually present from the onset of sexual life, four of their 17 men developed the disorder after a specific psychosexually traumatic event and only one of the remainder had ever previously ejaculated intravaginally.

Kaplan considers that the secondary form of retarded ejaculation is more common than Masters and Johnson believed, and Cooper considers that retarded ejaculation is a step in the direction towards erectile failure. Clearly it is important, from the therapeutic point of view, to distinguish between a primary form of the dysfunction resulting from severe sexual inhibition, and a secondary form which is more likely to occur when stimulation from the partner is insufficient and sexual interest flags.

General sexual and orgasmic dysfunction

As already stated, Kaplan distinguishes general sexual dysfunction from orgasmic dysfunction and considers that a woman may fail to be sexually aroused and yet experience an orgasm during intercourse. This possibility seems rather dubious although its reverse, i.e. the failure to reach orgasm in spite of sexual arousal, is certainly possible and indeed common. It may be regarded as the female equivalent of absent ejaculation in the male. It is probably better to consider the two forms of dysfunction together whilst recognizing that the arousal, plateau, and orgasmic phases are separate components of the female sexual response.

The primary and total form of general sexual dysfunction will usually be the result either of severe psychosexual inhibition or of a marked variation of sexual orientation, usually homosexuality. It is therefore essential to know whether the woman can ever become aroused under any circumstances. All writers agree that the woman requires a higher degree of emotional investment in her sexual partner than does the man, in order to become sexually aroused. Therefore, the secondary and situational forms of the dysfunction are likely to result from a disorder of basic relationship and attitudes to the partner. Resentment, hostility, contempt, and many other combinations of adverse attitudes to her partner are all sufficient causes of the dysfunction, although on occasion the woman may be able to abandon herself to sexual pleasure in spite of such attitudes.

In the absence of strong adverse attitudes the woman may fail to become aroused to the point of orgasm as a result of poor sexual technique. This may be due to the failure of the man to spend sufficient time in foreplay or to his own sexual difficulties and anxieties communicating to his partner and producing a failure of sexual reponse. For instance the partner of a man with premature ejaculation will seldom reach orgasm during intercourse and, owing to his nervousness, she will seldom be aroused at all. Masters and Johnson noted that the premature ejaculator generally arrives in the psychosexual clinic as a result of his wife's insistence. Kaplan also dispels the popular belief that the partner of the man with retarded or absent ejaculation enjoyes multiple orgasms whilst her partner is striving to reach one. She points out that the man's anxiety about his performance communicates to her, with resulting orgasmic failure on her part.

The actual position the couple adopt for intercourse may be the chief cause of orgasmic dysfunction in the woman. At one time, a distinction was drawn between 'clitoral' and 'vaginal' orgasm and the woman who only reported the clitoral variety was considered to be in deep psychological trouble. However, Masters and Johnson have dispelled that belief and shown that orgasm is a general bodily response but dependent upon clitoral stimulation. The position for intercourse frequently adopted is probably the 'male superior position' in which the couple are face to face with the man on top. This may have several disadvantages for the woman. She may feel psychologically powerless (which may or may not be a sexually arousing experience for her); she may feel physically uncomfortable, even to the point of feeling suffocated. Finally, as Kaplan points out, it is the position in which pubic pressure and clitoral stimulation is least likely to occur.

There is one cause of libidinal, and hence orgasmic, failure which must never be overlooked, and this is depressive illness. Libidinal failure is a common symptom of depressive illness. However, it is easy to overlook, for the depressive state may be quite mild or atypical and the loss of libido causes so much alarm and concern that the patient fails to mention other symptoms which may give a lead to the correct diagnosis. It is therefore the therapist's responsibility to conduct a careful examination of the mental state to establish, or rule out, the possibility of depressive illness *for there can be no greater error in the whole field of psychosexual therapy* than to subject a couple to needless and futile conjoint marital therapy when what is required to correct the disorder is effective antidepressive therapy.

Libidinal failure may first commence during a depressive illness but then persist after other symptoms of the state have remitted. This may often be the explanation for those long-standing states of libidinal failure which originally commenced following childbirth. Commencing in the setting of a mild and perhaps unrecognized puerperal depression the libidinal failure persists after other evidence of the disorder has abated. Why this should be so is not known. The phenomenon may have its basis in some persisting biophysical disorder affecting the neural centres which control sexual drive. However, an alternative explanation is that sexual confidence, and hence sexual response, is very susceptible to persistence once established. The damage occurs during the depressive phase and may persist unless carefully restored by a sensitive partner. It is good practice to carry out some preventative work in this area. A woman suffering from a depressive illness should be informed that libidinal failure is to be expected but that she may look forward with confidence to its restoration after recovery from the illness. If both she and her husband receive this explanation for the decline in sexual interest then the experience of it is less alarming to both of them and chain reactions of adverse attitudes and expectations may be avoided.

Vaginismus

In this condition the attempted passage of any object into the vagina leads to involuntary spasm of the muscles surrounding the vaginal inlet thus hindering or preventing further passage. As a result, penetration by the penis is difficult or quite impossible and likewise the insertion of tampons, pelvic examination, and even the attempt by the woman to insert her own finger into her vagina produce varying degrees of muscular spasm accompanied by anxiety. The condition may lead to the total impossibility of sexual intercourse but in less severe degrees partial penetration may be achieved accompanied by some perivaginal muscular spasm, anxiety, and discomfort. Masters and Johnson stated that the disorder cannot be diagnosed without a pelvic examination and thereby implied that if this is possible without general anaesthesia then the woman does not suffer from vaginismus; however, this all-or-nothing view does not allow for lesser degrees of severity of the condition. Moreover, in milder cases the woman may be able to tolerate pelvic examination with relative ease whilst being completely unable to allow penetration by the penis; probably the reverse situation also occurs.

Vaginismus arises on the basis of fear, guilt, embarrassment, the expectation of pain, and sometimes sheer aversion to the sexual act, in various combinations and degrees. Sometimes the condition is viewed in a relatively simplistic light as being a straightforward conditioned reflex and although this aspect may be nearer to the truth than a formulation based upon 'penis envy' resulting in a repressed wish to castrate the partner, in vaginismus, as in all sexual dysfunctions, the formulation of the case must rest upon a thorough assessment of all the factors operating in the production of the symptom.

In many cases there is a history of a prior psychotraumatic episode, which seemed to herald the onset of the condition. In one of the earliest descriptions of the condition, the author (Malleson, 1942) found that: 'The women had been, during infancy, conditioned to expect pain in the pelvic region by a foreign body, the offending object usually being the enema, the suppository or the old-fashioned soapstick so much employed in Victorian nurseries for the treatment of constipation.' With the passing of parental horror at the absence of the child's daily stool it is less likely that such a cause is to be found today; more common is the history of a premature attempt at intercourse by an embarrassed and frightened young girl which ended in pain and humiliation. Such a history of a psychotraumatic episode is not always found and in some cases more profound factors play a role, such as a deep-seated but unadmitted aversion to heterosexual intercourse in a homosexual woman who has attempted to enter upon a heterosexual relationship. Fear of pregnancy does not appear to be a frequent causative factor and indeed it is often a wish for a child which finally leads the woman to request treatment. The condition may appear, after previously normal sexual functioning, following a difficult labour with perineal bruising or tearing or an episode or vaginal infection which led to a period of painful intercourse (dyspareunia).

In some cases of vaginismus the woman's libidinal arousal and need for orgasmic experiences may be normal so that she and her partner engage upon a sexual relationship based upon mutual masturbation; at times this practice may satisfy both partners and it seems probable that women with a primary vaginismus should select partners who are sexually undemanding and easily satisfied. However, it is not possible to make any dogmatic statements about the condition for it is certain that those women who request treatment and are therefore seen by doctors, or other counsellors such as marriage guidance workers, represent only a proportion and a biassed sample of all women with vaginismus. However, for those women who do come for treatment it is likely that Ellison's (1968) observation that there was a background of ignorance and misinformation in 90 per cent of her hundred cases, can fairly be considered to apply to the population of women suffering from vaginismus.

TREATMENT OF PSYCHOSEXUAL DYSFUNCTION

In 1976 a Leading Article in the *British Medical Journal* stated: 'The "new sex therapy" has become a therapeutic vogue, big business in the United States with a growing demand in Britain. As with other forms of treatment, particularly those based upon psychological mechanisms, requests for it and the optimism of therapists have leaped ahead of real evidence of its effectiveness.' This distinctly cautious, if not frankly unenthusiastic, view could have been applied to the vast number of medical and surgical treatments that have arisen since man's first attempts to intervene against disease. None the less it is reproduced here in order to underline the need for detached appraisal of the results of treatment. The paper by Wright, Perreault, and Mathieu (1977) offers such an appraisal and guidelines for future research into therapy.

In place of the long-term psychoanalytic therapy, available to only a few, the introduction of the behavioural therapies by Wolpe (1958) and the later development of the two-week therapeutic programme by Masters and Johnson (1970) has led to the possibility of help for many more people. Wright and his colleagues conclude that, contrary to the predictions of many psychodynamic therapists, the short term 'directive' therapeutic techniques may sometimes be effective with certain selected patients but they also hold the opinion that at present no strong claims for the overall effectiveness of the directive therapies can be upheld.

The successful sex therapist must have at his disposal a wide range of therapeutic techniques and a competent understanding of the patient's or couple's whole problem. Only if these requirements are present can the danger of mismatching the therapy to the patient be avoided. Educative measures, directive and interpretive psychotherapy, conjoint marital therapy, behavioural therapy, drug therapy (and sometimes the stopping of drug therapy), methods to increase self-confidence, and treatment of other coexisting psychopathology will all have their place. The therapist must also possess the wisdom and experience to know when not to attempt treatment which may result in more misery and anxiety than any result may justify.

Few will doubt that the compendious work of Masters and Johnson has represented a real advance, resting as it does on the principles of involving both partners in the therapeutic plan, facilitation of open sexual communication, prescription of graded sexual tasks, and sexual education. The significance of their report of an overall success rate of 80 per cent, with 75 per cent remaining satisfied with the outcome after five years, may be in doubt; it may also be doubted that such success can be achieved in the absence of the dual therapist team, surrogate partners for single patients, a residential programme of two weeks away from the pressures of home and work, and patients highly selected for strong motivation and the absence of other serious psychopathology. Nevertheless the principles of education, self-awareness, understanding of the partner's problems and feelings, and reduction of sexual anxiety are unlikely to be reversed and represent a permanent advance in this field of therapy.

A brief description of the therapeutic programme is in place here since it represents an ideal to be aimed at even although cotherapists, daily interviews, and residential treatment may be unobtainable in many areas where sex therapy is practised. The initial interviews are carried out separately; the male cotherapist sees the man and the female cotherapist the woman. A full history is taken with assessment of attitudes and this is followed by a physical examination. Both partners are informed that they should not attempt to have intercourse until instructed to do so and this is essential information for a couple who would not otherwise know what was expected of them; it also has the immediate effect of reducing sexual anxiety which has probably been built up over a long period of repeated attempts and failure.

On the next day there is a round-table discussion with both partners and therapists present; the therapists then sum up their understanding of the problem and the relationship and invite comments and corrections from the partners. 'Homework' is then set and the basis of this is the training in sensate focus; in keeping with the principle aim of reducing sexual anxiety this is essentially non-demanding and non-threatening and instructions are given that between sessions with the cotherapists the couple should lie together naked and one should gently touch the other, at first avoiding the genitalia; the other partner may move the hand of the partner to indicate where he or she likes to be touched or stroked. As these tasks proceed there is a gradual acceptance of increasing erotic arousal but the therapists will withhold instructions to commence intercourse until there is evidence that arousal is strong and persistent and all parts of the body can be fondled by the other partner without inducing anxiety. During the sensate focus or 'pleasuring' sessions the person receiving the pleasuring must participate actively by putting his or her hand over the hand of the giving partner to indicate what causes pleasure.

Particular aspects of the therapeutic programme apply to specific dysfunctions. In the management of premature ejaculation the woman produces an erection of the penis by stroking it and the man signals when he feels he is reaching the point where ejaculation becomes inevitable. At this signal she firmly squeezes the shaft of the penis between her finger and thumb, the effect of which is that the man loses his erection and fails to ejaculate. This may be repeated several times in a session and later the man is encouraged to insert the penis into the vagina but he and his partner refrain from thrusting and may withdraw, reduce the erection, and again insert until confidence is built up that he has some control over the time he will take to ejaculate.

In vaginismus the man is invited to be present at the physical examination of his partner and to experience the perivaginal muscular spasm by inserting his finger a little way into the vaginal orifice. In the 'homework' sessions the couple are instructed to use a vaginal dilator, the woman first inserting it for herself and then instructing the partner to cover her hand with his while she does so.

An important aspect of the programme of therapy is the 'sanction' given by the therapists to the couple to behave in certain ways. This sanction has a powerful effect in helping to remove inhibitions and guilty feelings which have accumulated over years and contributed forcefully to the initiation and maintenance of the sexual dysfunction.

The therapeutic programme of Masters and Johnson did not appear fully fledged. It was based on their extensive prior study of the physiology of the sexual response and certain aspects of it were probably based upon the reported experience of other therapists. For instance, the technique for the management of premature ejaculation closely parallels a therapy advised by an American urological surgeon (Semans, 1956) fourteen years before the publication of *Human sexual inadequacy*. Wolpe (1958), in his classic work *Psychotherapy by reciprocal inhibition*, had also described the treatment of sexual dysfunction by the technique of systematic desensitization. Friedman (1962) had described a brief psychotherapeutic approach for non-consummation carried out by doctors working in family planning based upon exploration of the women's fantasies; these doctors reported their experiences in group sessions led by a psychiatrist working on the principles laid down by Balint; of those with a known outcome 81 per cent succeeded in consummating their marriage.

The role of the administration of synthetic hormones requires more extensive investigation than it has yet received. There have been very few published reports indicating that the administration of androgens to the male suffering from sexual dysfunction is a successful venture and it seems more likely that they have a limited but definite therapeutic effect in the female suffering from a diminution of sexual arousal in the absence of specific relationship problems. Carney, Bancroft, and Mathews (1978) found that sublingual testosterone was effective in enhancing sexual arousability in women. In a reply to that report, Snaith and Jardine (1979) considered that there might be an adverse effect of this hormone on the foetus if the women were to become pregnant and it was as yet too early to advise the widespread use of such therapy without the most stringent precautions against pregnancy occurring whilst the drug is being taken.

Therapy for sexual dysfunction is still in its infancy and much remains to be done in assessing the effectiveness of different treatments and combinations of treatment in different aspects of sexual dysfunction and the wider field of disturbance of the marital relationship. The latter aspect is an even more nebulous concept and harder to assess but an attempt has been made by Crowe (1978) who found that in conjoint marital therapy a directive approach appeared to be more efficacious on most measures than either an interpretive or a supportive (control) approach to therapy.

The elicitation of prognostic factors with various therapeutic approaches is an area which will require much attention but an initial contribution to this area of study has been made by Munjack and Kanno (1977) who have reviewed the published accounts of treatment of sexual dysfunction in women. Among their conclusions, those with the highest rank were: (a) that high levels of sexual anxiety are indicative of an unfavourable prognosis when methods other than systematic desensitization are used; (b) that behavioural approaches utilizing educational and retraining procedures and other strategies based on learning principles have substantially improved treatment results of female sexual inhibition, while shortening therapy time in patients selected for the absence of pervasive psychological disturbance.

Good prognostic pointers for therapeutic intervention in sexual dysfunction will depend upon many factors related to the attitude of the therapist to the patient and confidence in the techniques used. So far as the outcome can be adjudged at initial evaluation of the problem, Cooper has described good prognostic pointers in the male (1970a) and female (1970b). The man is likely to have referred himself or the referral has resulted from a frank discussion between both partners. He will be married and under the age of thirty years and will have developed an acute dysfunction in response to stress. His heterosexual interest remains strong as evidenced by continuing masturbation to orgasm though his preferred outlet is heterosexual coitus. He will have a good relationship with his wife who is willing to co-operate in the treatment programme. The good prognostic points for the woman are broadly the same; the duration of the dysfunction is short and has occurred after a period of normal sexual function; her preferred outlet is heterosexual coitus and her attitude to her male partner is affectionate; there is no gross abnormality of personality and she has no marked abhorrence of her own or her partner's genitalia; she herself has initiated the referral for treatment.

References

ANSARI, J. M. A. (1975). A study of 65 impotent males. *Br. J. Psychiat.* **127**, 337–42.
*—— (1976). Impotence: prognosis (a controlled study). *Br. J. Psychiat.* **128**, 194–9.
*BANCROFT, J. (1977). Hormones and sexual behaviour. *Psychol. Med.* **7**, 553–6.
BORS, E. and COMARR, E. (1960). Neurological disturbance of sexual dysfunction with special reference to 529 patients with spinal cord injury. *Urol. Surv.* **10**, 191–222.
British Medical Journal (1975). The elderly testis. Leading article. *Br. med. J.* **iii**, 2–3.

—— (1976). Treatment of erectile impotence. Leading article. *Br. med. J.* **ii**, 1298–9.

—— (1978). Endocrine basis for sexual dysfunction. Leading article. *Br. med. J.* **iv**, 1516–17.

BULPITT, C. J. and DOLLERY, C. T. (1973). Side-effects of hypotensive agents evaluated by a self-administered questionnaire. *Br. med. J.* **iii**, 485–90.

CARNEY, A., BANCROFT, J., and MATHEWS, A. (1978). Combination of hormonal and psychological treatment for female sexual unresponsiveness. *Br. J. Psychiat.* **133**, 339–46.

COOPER, A. J. (1969). Clinical and therapeutic studies in premature ejaculation. *Comp. Psychiat.* **10**, 285–95.

*—— (1970a). Guide to treatment and short-term prognosis of male potency disorders in hospital and general practice. *Br. med. J.* **i**, 157–9.

*—— (1970b). Frigidity, treatment and short-term prognosis. *J. Psychosomat. Res.* **14**, 133–47.

—— (1972). Diagnosis and management of endocrine impotence. *Br. med. J.* **ii**, 34–6.

—— ISMAIL, A. A., SMITH, C. G., and LORAINE, J. A. (1970). Androgen function in 'psychogenic' and 'constitutional' types of impotence. *Br. med. J.* **iii**, 17–20.

*CROWE, M. J. (1978). Conjoint marital therapy: a controlled study. *Psychol. Med.* **8**, 623–36.

ELLENBERG, M. (1971). Impotence in diabetes: the neurological factor. *Ann. int. Med.* **75**, 313–19.

ELLISON, C. (1968). Psychosomatic factors in unconsummated marriage. *J. Psychosomat. Res.* **12**, 61–5.

FAERMAN, I., GLOVER, L., FOX, D., JADZINSKI, M. N., and RAPAPORT, M. (1974). Impotence and diabetes. *Diabetes* **23**, 971–6.

FOX, C. A., ISMAIL, A. A., LOVE, D. N., KIRKHAM, K., and LORAINE, J. A. (1972). Studies of the relationship of plasma testosterone to human sexual activity. *J. Endocr.* **45**, 145.

FRIEDMAN, L. J. (1962). *Virgin wives; a study of unconsummated marriages*. Mind and Medicine Monography. Tavistock, London.

GORER, G. (1971). *Sex and marriage in England today*. Nelson, London.

HASTINGS, D. (1963). *Impotence and frigidity*. Little, Brown and Company, Boston.

HIERONS, R. and SAUNDERS, M. (1966). Impotence in patients with temporal lobe lesions. *Lancet* **ii**, 761–3.

JOHNSON, J. (1965a). Sexual impotence and the limbic system. *Br. J. Psychiat.* **111**, 300–3.

—— (1965b). Androgyny and disorders of sexual potency. *Br. med. J.* **ii**, 572–3.

JONES, H. G. (1976). The psychology of sex. In *Psychosexual problems* (ed. H. Milne and S. J. Hardy). Crosby Lockwood Staples, London.

KAPLAN, H. S. (1974). *The new sex therapy*. Ballière Tindall, London.

KINSEY, A. C., POMEROY, W. B., and MARTIN, C. E. (1948). *Sexual behaviour in the human male*. Saunders, Philadelphia.

————— (1953). *Sexual behaviour in the human female.* Saunders, Philadelphia.

KOLODNY, R. C. (1971). Sexual dysfunction in diabetic females. *Diabetes* **20**, 557–9.

—— KAHN, C. B., GOLDSTEIN, H. H., and BARNETT, D. M. (1974). Sexual function in the diabetic man. *Diabetes* **23**, 306–9.

LENNOX, W. G. and LENNOX, H. A. (1960). *Epilepsy and related disorders*, Vol. I. Churchill, London.

MALLESON, J. (1942). Vaginismus: its management and psychogenesis. *Br. med. J.* **ii**, 213–16.

MASTERS, W. and JOHNSON, V. (1966). *The human sexual response.* Little, Brown and Company, Boston.

—— —— (1970). *Human sexual inadequacy.* Little, Brown and Company, Boston.

MUNJACK, D. J. and KANNO, P. H. (1977). Prognosis in the treatment of female sexual inhibition. *Comp. Psychiat.* **18**, 481–8.

MUNRO, D., HORNE, H. W., and PAULL, D. P. (1948). The effect of injury to the spinal cord and cauda equina on sexual potency of men. *New Engl. J. Med.* **239**, 903–11.

RENSHAW, D. C. (1975). Impotence in diabetics. *Dis. nerv. Syst.* **36**, 369–71.

RUBIN, A. and BABBOTT, D. (1958). Impotence and diabetes. *J. Am. med. Ass.* **168**, 498–500.

SCHAPIRO, B. (1947). Premature ejaculation. *J. Urol.* **50**, 374–9.

SCHOFIELD, M. (1973). *The sexual behaviour of young adults.* Allen Lane, London.

SEGRAVES, R. T. (1977). Pharmacological agents causing sexual dysfunction. *J. Sex Marit. Ther.* **3**, 157–76.

SEMANS, J. H. (1956). Premature ejaculation, a new approach. *Sth. med. J. Nashville* **49**, 353–8.

SILVER, J. R. (1975). Sexual problems in disorders of the nervous system. *Br. med. J.* **iii**, 480–2.

—— and OWENS, E. (1975). Sexual disorders in disorders of the nervous system: psychological reactions. *Br. med. J.* **iii**, 532–4.

SNAITH, R. P. and JARDINE, M. Y. (1979). Androgens in sexual dysfunction: a plea for caution. *Br. J. Psychiat.* **134**, 447.

TALBOT, H. S. (1949). A report on the sexual function of paraplegics. *J. Urol.* **61**, 265–70.

UDREY, J. R. and MORRIS, N. W. (1968). Distribution of coitus in the menstrual cycle. *Nature, Lond.* **220**, 593.

WEISSMAN, M. M. and SLABEY, A. E. (1973). Oral contraceptives and psychiatric disturbance. *Br. J. Psychiat.* **123**, 513–18.

WOLPE, J. (1958). Psychotherapy by reciprocal inhibition. Stanford University Press, California.

*WRIGHT, J., PERREAULT, R., and MATHIEU, M. (1977). The treatment of sexual dysfunction. *Archs gen. Psychiat.* **34**, 881–90.

ZEITLIN, A. B., COTTRELL, T., and LLOYD, F. A. (1957). Sexology of the paraplegic male. *J. Fert. Steril.* **8**, 337–44.

7

Anxiety control training: a psychotherapeutic technique

PSYCHOTHERAPEUTIC techniques continue to multiply and today there are available a vast number from which the aspiring therapist is invited to make his choice. Many of them bear the individual stamp of the author but few of them are really original and, whether or not the acknowledgement is explicitly made, nearly all the 'new' techniques have evolved from older therapeutic approaches to human distress. Frank (1977) has suggested that some of these systems belong to the 'religio-magical' tradition in which expectant faith is clearly the operative factor, whereas others present 'scientific' credentials even though the scientific laws on which they are founded are not always open to the process of testing and refutation. Some systems, such as Primal Scream Therapy, bear emotive titles but others, such as Systematic Rational Restructuring, are couched in the more sober terms of logical thought. Elsewhere, Frank (1974; 1976) has drawn the conclusion that, central to all psychotherapeutic systems, is the process of combating the personal sense of demoralization by increasing the individual's awareness of his own mastery over his environment. Bandura (1977) has used the phrase 'self-efficacy' in place of mastery.

Some psychotherapeutic systems seek to relieve the distress of the individual by providing him with insight into the supposed cause of his disorder, others encourage him to alter his attitudes towards himself and his environment, yet others foster a sense of higher purpose transcending present misery whilst others seek to teach the individual self-control over his turbulent emotions. Certainly there is a growing demand for psychotherapy, at least within the Western world, and with this increase in demand has come the requirement that techniques should be more rapidly effective in relieving distress; the place of the leisurely system of psychoanalysis in the setting of the National Health Service has been questioned (Shepherd, 1979).

The system of psychotherapy described here belongs to what today is usually called the cognitive-behavioural group of therapies. It has emerged in a somewhat piecemeal fashion from a variety of sources during two decades of clinical application in a health service setting; the pressure of numbers of patients requiring help dictates that few patients can receive more than six to eight hours of individual therapeutic time so that any technique must be expected to be effective for a high proportion of patients within the limits of that time. As with many psychotherapeutic techniques Anxiety Control Training has not yet been subjected to a critical investigation of its effectiveness and at this stage the writer can only state that, with careful selection of patients, the results are excellent or good in about two thirds after 15–20 twenty-minute weekly sessions and of the remaining patients, many derive some degree of benefit. The technique is certainly not a panacea for all psychiatric disorder and the requirements for a successful outcome are first that the disorder is based upon anxiety and secondly that the patient is sufficiently well motivated to devote personal effort to bringing about his own improvement; given these two requirements the technique is applicable to about five per cent of patients referred to an average psychiatric clinic. Before the details of procedure are presented some of the background to the development of this approach to psychotherapy will be examined.

Anxiety Control Training (ACT) has its roots in meditational practice and particularly that form called Autogenic Training, introduced by Schultz in the 1920s. In the 1930s Jacobson introduced the technique of Progressive Relaxation: whilst this system was welcomed by Yates (1946) it was also criticized for its concentration on technique to the neglect of the attitudes and particular problems of the patient. In her Association Set technique, Yates introduced into the setting of the relaxation procedure: 'Explanation, confidence-building, motivation, self-direction and specific objectives'. Specifically, the patient was taught to associate a sense of calm with a specific word or phrase which he could repeat to himself at times of stress, a 'device to meet emergencies and critical emotional situations'.

In 1958 Wolpe reported his technique of systematic desensitization in *Psychotherapy by reciprocal inhibition*. This work, which had its roots in behaviourism, gave a powerful stimulus to the growing interest in psychotherapeutic techniques based on learning theory which were to be gathered together under the rubric of behaviour therapy. The history of the development of behavioural techniques into cognitive therapies has been traced by Mahoney (1974) who pointed out that, whereas the early behaviour modifiers restricted their operations to observable phenomena there was a fast-growing discontent with the persistence in ignoring private, or covert, events and especially attitudes, self-concepts, and beliefs.

Two concepts which began to emerge in the 1960s were those of 'self-control' and 'induced anxiety' and both these concepts have helped to shape the psychotherapeutic technique presented here. Cautela (1969) summarized the early application of self-control within a behavioural therapy framework; he referred to the work of Ferster, Goldiamond, and Homme together with his own Covert Sensitization technique whereby the individual plays a major part in his own treatment by producing in fantasy both the maladaptive response and the aversive consequence. Cautela concluded that the teaching of self-control involved:

> 1. Providing the individual with responses he can initiate, whenever necessary, to change the probability of undesirable responses.
> 2. Instructing the individual when, and under what conditions, to make the self-controlling response.

He pointed out the advantages of self-control techniques, in that more conditioning trials could occur within a given time interval, thus shortening the time spent in therapy; also that further maladaptive behaviour could be prevented by not allowing undesirable responses to increase in strength.

The introduction of induced anxiety into the psychotherapeutic scene was described by Sipprelle (1967) who recognized that his technique combined elements of the two different approaches of Wolpe and of Stampfl. In this procedure no attempt is made to get the individual to re-experience specific traumatic incidents, as in the older technique of abreaction; under hypnosis, the individual is instructed to turn his attention inward and to experience steadily increasing uncomfortable emotions of fear and anxiety but no specific suggestions as to the source of the anxiety are made; the occurrence of overt emotional disturbance is then countered by suggestions of calm and the session is terminated with a strong suggestion that the individual will continue to feel calm and relaxed. A similar procedure was later developed by Meichenbaum (1977) in his technique of 'stress inoculation'.

Goldfried (1971) interpreted the therapeutic effects of systematic desensitization in terms of the acquirement of self-control. In accordance with this view, desensitization is considered to be a process whereby the individual acquires a skill in reducing anxiety which then enables him to exercise a greater degree of self-control in a variety of anxiety-provoking situations and not merely the specific situation to which he was being desensitized. The major change of emphasis is from the technique as practised by the therapist to the skill acquired by the individual. Goldfried pointed out that the following procedural modifications to the process of desensitization were required by his model:

1. The individual is informed that the therapeutic sessions provide practice in overcoming anxiety and are in fact a rehearsal of what he will eventually learn to do for himself.

2. the relaxation training enables the perception of the proprioceptive feedback of anxiety;

3. there is less need for the presentation of anxiety imagery in a strictly hierarchical order as the individual uses the sessions to learn to cope with anxiety in general rather than anxiety associated with specific situations;

4. in the procedure of systematic desensitization the individual is informed that he should eliminate the anxiety image as soon as he feels anxious but, in the modification, this instruction is not given and instead he is encouraged to maintain the experience of anxiety for longer periods of time before controlling it.

In a review of the concept of behaviour therapy as a process of developing self-control, Gelder (1979) has underlined many important points relevant to psychotherapeutic techniques. He points out that many psychiatric patients would like to play a more effective part in their own treatment but clinicians have traditionally neglected these aspirations; since they believe the main thrust of the therapeutic effect takes place in the treatment sessions, less attention is paid to what occurs between sessions. Although there has been an emphasis on the self-regulatory aspects of behaviour therapy for over a decade the actual application of self-control procedures has remained rather narrow. Gelder remarks that it is surprising that behaviour therapists have paid so little attention to the problem of ensuring that their patients understand what they should attempt to do between sessions and he draws attention to the value of the self-instructional pamphlet which can be given to the patient. Meichenbaum (1977) has also pointed out that when behaviour therapy is augmented by a self-instructional package then greater treatment efficacy, more generalization and greater persistence of treatment effects are obtained. A further important point from Gelder's paper is the need to provide the patient with a counter-neurotic device which is sufficiently simple for him to practice on his own and yet sufficiently effective to have a perceptible impact in reducing emotional distress. This, of course, is the key to all self-control procedures.

Meichenbaum introduced a more definite cognitive element into behavioural psychotherapy and emphasized the modification of the patient's 'internal language', that is his expectations of inevitable emotional consequences following upon encounter with certain situations. The most important of these techniques is that of 'coping imagery' in which, during the treatment sessions, the patient is instructed to visualize himself coping with stress; as a result of this procedure he is more likely to regard the experience of anxiety as having a beneficial aspect since it enables him to rehearse his developing skill in controlling it. Meichenbaum concluded that the cognitive-coping approach to desensitization illustrates that the standard desensitization approach can be successfully modified and supplemented by treatment procedures designed to change the client's self-labelling and cognitive processes.

In a review of the effects of coping-skills training for the management of anxiety, Barrios and Shigetomi (1979) noted the growing interest in these techniques but also pointed to the relative dearth of information concerning their efficacy in clinical settings, for most of the originators of the variety of procedures have carried out the evaluation in such non-clinical groups as test-anxious students. They concluded that there was evidence for the efficacy of these techniques but called for more investigation into their effects on clinical groups and also for an examination of the preventive aspects of coping-skills training.

The clinical psychotherapeutic technique of Anxiety Control Training was first briefly presented some years ago (Snaith, 1974) but since that time it has undergone modification in the light of both the theoretical advances just reviewed and further clinical evaluation. Essentially it is a technique through which the patient acquires the skill of emotional self-control and is encouraged in the process of cognitive reshaping of destructive or maladaptive attitudes towards himself and his environment. The procedure of ACT may only be expected to be successful when the patient is well motivated to make a positive contribution towards his own improvement or recovery and secondly it is likely to be beneficial only when anxiety is the basis of the disorder. Patients with a biologically based affective disorder will not benefit from the procedure, even though the most prominent symptoms of the disorder are those of anxiety; however, residual anxiety symptomatology following effective treatment of the affective disorder may be improved although the therapeutic process should be monitored for the recurrence of depressive symptomatology which will slow down or negate further progress.

THE TECHNIQUE OF ANXIETY CONTROL TRAINING (ACT)

1. Explanation and preparation

Having decided that the patient's disorder might respond to ACT the therapist explains the procedure in some detail. It is pointed out that the acquisition of skill in controlling anxiety is dependent upon regular practice and in this way it is similar to learning any other skill, such as mastery of a foreign language or proficiency in a sport. The outcome will be entirely dependent upon the patient's application to the procedure and the basis of this is autohypnotic (or meditative) practice conducted regularly for ten minutes twice a day. He is informed that this practice may be a little difficult at first until he 'gets the hang' of the technique but that the weekly sessions with the therapist will enable him to practice it with increasing facility. He should be advised not to expect immediate results but that he will probably notice, after some weeks, that situations which used to cause him distress do so to a lesser extent and at that stage his increasing self-confidence will lead to more rapid progress.

Some therapists may not wish to employ the terms hypnosis and autohypnosis because they reject what they regard as their arcane overtones and for this reason they may decide to use a more popular phrase such as 'relaxation training'. This is acceptable so long as the patient is not misled by the everyday use of the word relaxation; he should understand that the procedure is one of quite intense mental concentration and is therefore the obverse of a ten-minute nap or doze. In fact care should be taken to stress that the autohypnotic sessions should not be attempted when the patient is very tired or has recently taken alcohol or a sedative drug.

At the end of the explanatory session the patient is given a pamphlet (reproduced on pp. 223–6) which explains the programme of therapy in simple terms and he is advised to read it carefully so that he can discuss any points which are not clear to him at the next session. Patients, even those who are well-motivated towards the procedure, frequently state that they find difficulty in putting aside the twice daily ten-minute sessions and this is especially the case with mothers of young children or people with irregular hours of work. They should be advised, before therapy commences, to organize their time and to try to get into the habit by simply going to a room where they can sit quietly on their own for the ten-minute periods. The pamphlet may also be shown to members of the patient's family so that their help and co-operation in this requirement can be enlisted.

2. The therapeutic sessions

At the first session the programme is again discussed and questions are answered. If the term 'hypnosis' is to be used the patient may be asked if he has any worries about such a procedure; he may think that he will be deprived of all personal control or, if his only acquaintance with hypnosis is that of stage entertainment, that he will be required to carry out extraordinary or humiliating feats. He may be assured that this is not the case, that he himself will carry out the hypnosis and that the therapist will only be there to guide him and facilitate the process. In order to underline the fact that the patient controls the procedure of hypnosis the therapist should avoid imposing a position, such as the requirement to lie on a couch, and the patient should be invited to choose his own position. Ideal for the purpose is a fully-upholstered chair which the patient may adjust for himself to his favoured position.

After the patient has found his comfortable position the therapist then takes a seat to one side from where he can carefully observe him. The particular format of the induction of hypnosis will be a matter of the personal style of the therapist, but the author has found the following to be generally acceptable and successful:

In the pamphlet it is clearly stated how the patient should bring a session to an end for himself. It is also stated that under no circumstances should the autohypnosis be attempted in any situation where a distraction of attention could cause danger, such as driving a vehicle or climbing a ladder; the patient's attention should be especially drawn to this paragraph before therapy commences.

4. Synthesis

After the third or fourth session the therapist should start to introduce anxiety imagery into the sessions. He should discuss this beforehand with the patient and inform him that on no account will the anxiety become more intense than he can control. At the same time a coping device to control anxiety is suggested. The session may go as follows:

> . . . now you are going to leave your calm scene and you are going to enter a scene where you will feel anxious . . . when you begin to feel anxious you will take three or four deep breaths and that will control your anxiety and enable you to stay in the scene without much discomfort . . . passing over to the anxiety scene now . . .
> [The therapist should now carefully observe the patient for the next minute or two. He may notice that either nothing happens—in which case it may be assumed that the patient has not been able to image himself in an anxiety scene—or he may notice that the patient shows visible signs of distress but no evidence of the coping mechanism; or he may notice distress followed by the deep breaths, in which case he can be assured that the patient is coping, or attempting to cope, with the anxiety correctly. In any case, the session should not be brought to an end without the following instruction:]
> . . . you are now returning to your calm scene and gaining complete control over anxiety . . . deep control. . . . Now we will bring the session to an end by counting back from six to one, when I reach one all the heaviness will have passed away but you will still be calm and relaxed . . . six, five, four, three, lighter and lighter, two and one.

As always, a careful note is made of the patient's report of his experience in the session. If no anxiety was experienced he may be informed that this is frequently the case at the first presentation of anxiety imagery and simply indicates that confidence in control over anxiety is not yet fully established but that this will occur in future sessions. In the case of unsuccessful self-control through the coping mechanism the patient may again be informed that this is also common in the early stages but that, with further practice, he will soon learn this control. In the case of successful self-control the patient is informed that, through the simple procedure of taking a few deep breaths he will eventually find that he can control anxiety for himself in real life circumstances.

For those patients who are unable to visualize either calm scenes or anxiety scenes the difficulty can be overcome by the therapist simply describing an anxiety provoking scene to the patient during the session, for example:

> . . . you now feel calm and relaxed but shortly you will feel rather anxious and you will control this anxiety by taking four, slow, deep breaths . . . you are now thinking about entering a room full of people, and some people stop talking and turn to look at you . . . [or whatever the situation is in which the patient generally experiences anxiety].

As the programme continues, and usually after the patient has experienced three or four anxiety-inducing sessions with the therapist, with successful self-control, he is encouraged to attempt to incorporate anxiety imagery into his own autohypnotic sessions. At each session a note is made of the patient's report of his success, or lack of success, with this procedure. Eventually, when all is going well, the patient will gain the confidence to experience increasing intensity of anxiety in his sessions in the certain knowledge that he can control it, and within a short time he will become aware that he is experiencing less anxiety in the real life circumstances which formerly caused him distress. Frequently, good progress has been made within twelve weekly sessions but of course some patients require more prolonged help.

It should be noted that the pace of the programme is largely controlled by the patient; no anxiety imagery is imposed upon him, but merely the suggestion of feeling anxious is introduced at an early stage. However, in the short discussion before each weekly session the therapist should enquire about progress and may sometimes consider that a certain amount of direction should be imposed; for instance, he may inform a travel phobic patient at a certain stage in the programme that he now considers the journey to the treatment centre could be made by bus. Many patients require and respond well to direction by the therapist whereas others manage well without it. An important part of the programme is the 'reward' for progress that has been made, for this helps to increase the patient's self-confidence which may still be in the nursling stage; the therapist should therefore not fail to take note of and reward progress with encouragement.

REASONS FOR FAILURE

As with all therapeutic procedures ACT will fail with a proportion of patients in spite of apparently favourable indications at the initial assessment. If no progress at all has been made after fifteen weeks there is usually little point in continuing with ACT and a careful reassessment of the case is required. Possible reasons for failure include lack of motivation, the occurrence of fresh adversities in the patient's life, 'sabotage' of the programme by the patient's spouse or family members (see the section on this topic in the chapter on *Anxiety and the phobic neuroses*) or the occurrence of a depressive state during the course of therapy.

Lack of motivation for change is perhaps the most common reason for failure of therapy and this may be present in spite of apparently good motivation at the initial assessment. The patient may be deriving too much secondary gain from his neurosis to really wish to recover from the disorder and he may have entered therapy simply as a façade to himself and to others. However, it should not automatically be assumed that all patients who make no progress are lacking in motivation for other factors may be operating or ACT may have been the incorrect choice of therapy in the first place.

Another important cause for failure of the therapy is that of an untreated, or unsuccessfully treated, affective disorder underlying the patient's symptoms (attention was called to this matter in Chapter 1). Depression may not have been present at the commencement of the therapy but may occur during therapy; this should not be considered to be 'symptom substitution' for many patients with anxiety-based neuroses frequently experience depressive episodes. A recurrence of an affective disorder should always be suspected in the case of the patient who has initially made good progress but who then complains that he is no longer able to concentrate upon his autohypnotic sessions. In the case of a temporary period of an affective disorder with prominent depressive symptomatology the ACT programme should be suspended, if only temporarily, until the affective disorder has been treated, if necessary with antidepressant drugs. Beck (1976) has pointed out that depressed patients experience distorted attitudes towards themselves which causes them to withhold self-reinforcement. Self-reinforcement is a process which is integral to the success of ACT.

The completion of the Irritability-Depression-Anxiety (IDA) Scale (Snaith *et al.*, 1978) at the initial assessment and at intervals throughout the therapy will be an aid to the detection of significant depressive symptomatology which would be likely to impede progress.

OTHER INDICATIONS FOR ACT

In general it may be said that ACT may be a successful form of brief psychotherapy for disorders based upon, and maintained by, anxiety. These include, not only the classical phobic neuroses, but also mild degrees of pervasive anxiety (a more severe degree of pervasive state anxiety is usually a manifestation of an affective disorder and will not respond to ACT). Social and sexual anxiety may be improved so long as ACT is undertaken in the setting of a full appraisal of the patient's circumstances and interpersonal relationships and, in the latter case, the involvement of the patient's partner will almost always be necessary (see Chapter 6). Some psychosomatic conditions such as tension headache and asthma aggravated by anxiety may be improved and Patel and North (1975) have shown that a similar therapeutic approach may help some patients whose hypertension is maintained largely by psychic factors. Longstanding personality disorder, with anxiety as the most prominent feature, may be improved but with such patients it is not reasonable to expect marked improvement in the short term.

Impulse control disorders such as exhibitionism may respond to an adaptation of ACT so long as there is good motivation to overcome the disorder. It should also be possible to adapt the programme to help with the control of certain obsessional symptoms. Addictive habits such as tobacco smoking may be helped and the writer has frequently treated patients for other disorders who have casually remarked at the end of successful therapy: 'By the way, I've stopped smoking.' There may be an occasional role for ACT in the management of well-motivated alcoholics.

Cognitive-behavioural therapies such as ACT are still at a very early stage of development and at present research into the outcome of all psychotherapeutic treatments is still gravely deficient. The role of such procedures in the total armamentarium of psychotherapy should be accorded priority in psychiatric research.

APPENDIX: An example of the manual to be given to the patient.

Anxiety Control Training

This pamphlet outlines a programme for learning self-control over anxiety. It has been used for many years and has been found to be a successful method. However, it is only successful for those who are prepared to make the effort to follow the rules and to put in the required practice every day. Whereas most medical treatments depend upon the skill of the doctor, Anxiety Control Training depends upon learning. To learn anything well, such as to play a musical instrument or a game, an instructor can show the rules but the person will only become proficient if he practises regularly. In Anxiety Control Training, your therapist (doctor or psychologist) can take you through the programme by easy steps and show you what to do at each stage but your eventual ability to control your own anxiety will depend upon yourself. So first make up your mind that you really wish to learn self-control over anxiety.

When you have made up your mind on that point let your therapist know and he will arrange for you to begin sessions which are usually carried out on a weekly basis. However, there may be a waiting time before the therapist can start the programme and there is something that you can begin to do straight away. That is to get yourself organized for your ten-minute practice sessions which you must carry out twice a day. A lot of people say they want to learn anxiety control but then have difficulty in finding the time for these daily sessions and, as a result, the method fails. It is really just a matter of organizing your time and getting into the habit of going to a room where you can be still and quiet for ten minutes twice a day. Busy people may find that they have to get up a bit earlier in the morning and mothers of young children may have to arrange to do their sessions at the time when their husbands are at home to look after the children. It is very important to arrange to do your sessions at times when you are not very tired for when you begin the programme you will discover that quite a lot of concentration is required and this is difficult to do if you are very tired. Some people who do the sessions after a day's work find that the best thing is to first have a brief rest and then carry out the session.

The only other absolute requirement for your practice sessions is that you should be in a room on your own for it is not possible to concentrate if other people are walking in and out of the room. Otherwise do not expect absolute quiet in the house for that is not necessary. Eventually you will learn to control your anxiety in everyday life and of course in everyday life there is always a lot of noise going on.

So, in order to organize your time and therefore to be ready to start anxiety control training, just go to a room on your own, find a comfortable position in a chair or lying on a bed, and be still for ten minutes twice a day.

When you commence your sessions with your therapist he will show you a way to concentrate your thoughts and become aware of the absence of tension. Every therapist has his own style of doing this but usually you will be asked to settle into a comfortable position and to concentrate your thoughts on his voice. He will then talk quietly about sensations you will be experiencing in your own body, your arms becoming heavy, quiet breathing, sinking back more deeply into the chair, and so on. It is always easier to achieve a feeling of deep relaxation under the guidance of a therapist than on your own for concentration on his voice will help you to stop your thoughts from wandering. Don't worry if you feel you have not achieved control over tension at the first session for many people find that it takes a few sessions in order to experience this.

Once you have experienced the state of absence of tension with the therapist you will find that it is easier for you to achieve the same state in your own daily practice sessions. In order to do this you will have to substitute your own thoughts for the therapist's voice. It is therefore very important that you should decide on the words which you are going to let run through your mind in your session. Every time your thoughts wander concentrate your mind again on the words of the exercise. A suitable form of words to begin with is:

I AM STILL – STILL AND BECOMING CALM – SINK-ING BACK INTO THE CHAIR – BECOMING CALM – AND STILL

At the end of every exercise which you do on your own you should bring the session to a definite conclusion by stretching your arms and legs and taking one or two deep breaths.

You may alter the words if you wish, but the important thing is to be quite clear just what words you are going to let run through your mind before you start the exercise. Some people find it helpful to read the

MEICHENBAUM, D. (1977). *Cognitive–behaviour modification: an integrative approach.* Plenum, New York.

PATEL, C. and NORTH, W. R. S. (1975). Randomized controlled trial of yoga and biofeedback in management of hypertension. *Lancet* **ii**, 93–5.

SHEPHERD, M. (1979). Psychoanalysis, psychotherapy and the health services. *Br. med. J.* **ii**, 1557–9.

SIPPRELLE, C. N. (1967). Induced anxiety. *Psychother. Theory, Res. Pract.* **4**, 36–40.

SNAITH, R. P. (1974). A method of psychotherapy based on relaxation techniques. *Br. J. Psychiat.* **124**, 473–81.

—— CONSTANTOPOULOS, A. A., JARDINE, M. Y., and McGUFFIN, P. (1978). A clinical scale for the self-assessment of irritability. *Br. J. Psychiat.* **132**, 164–71.

WOLPE, J. (1958). *Psychotherapy by reciprocal inhibition.* Stanford University Press, California.

YATES, D. H. (1946). Relaxation in psychotherapy. *J. gen. Psychol.* **34**, 213–38.

Index